BODYMIND

Also by Ken Dychtwald

Millennium: Glimpses into the 21st Century (with A. Villoldo)
The Keys to a High Performance Lifestyle
Wellness and Health Promotion for the Elderly
The Role of the Hospital in an Aging Society:
  A Blueprint for Action (with M. Zitter)
Age Wave

BODYMIND

BY

KEN DYCHTWALD

With illustrations by Juan Barberis,
Jad King, and Amy Hosa

JEREMY P. TARCHER, INC.
Los Angeles

For
my mother, father, and brother,
who enfold me with their love, honesty,
and dignity

Library of Congress Cataloging-in-Publication Data

Dychtwald, Ken, 1950–
    Bodymind.

    Reprint. Originally published: New York : Pantheon Books, ©1977.
    Bibliography: p. 279
    Includes index.
    1. Mind and body.   I. Title.
[BF161.D9   1986]   616.89   86-658
ISBN 0-87477-375-X

Jeremy P. Tarcher, Inc., 5858 Wilshire Blvd., Los Angeles, CA 90036

Grateful acknowledgment is made to the following for permission to reprint previously published material:

E. P. Dutton & Co., Inc.: For excerpts from pp. 1–4 of *Cosmic Consciousness*, by
R. M. Bucke. Copyright 1901, 1923 by E. P. Dutton & Co., Inc.

M. Evans & Co., Inc., For excerpts from pp. 14–16 of *Body Language*, by Julius
Fast. Copyright © 1970 by Julius Fast.

Harper & Row Publishers, Inc.: For excerpts from pp. 65, 77, 78, 79, 81, 85, 86,
and 194 of *Here Comes Everybody*, by William C. Schutz. Copyright © 1971 by
William C. Schutz.

Prentice-Hall, Inc.: For excerpt from pp. 160–2 of *The Nature of Personal Reality*,
by Jane Roberts. Copyright © 1974 by Jane Roberts.

Random House, Inc., and The Bookworks: For excerpts from pp. 202–3 and
illustration by Joseph Jaqua from p. 30 of *Total Orgasm*, by Jack Lee Rosenberg,
illustrated by Joseph Jaqua. Copyright © 1973 by Jack Lee Rosenberg.

Manufactured in the United States of America

CONTENTS

List of Illustrations   vii

Preface   ix

Acknowledgments   xiii

Foreword   xv

1 BODY/MIND   3

2 OVERVIEW   18

3 FEET AND LEGS   47

4 PELVIS   79

5 ABDOMINAL REGION AND
   LOWER BACK   119

6 CHEST CAVITY   144

7 SHOULDERS AND ARMS   163

8 NECK, THROAT, AND JAW   186

9 FACE AND HEAD   216

10 BODYMIND   256

Notes   265
Bibliography   279
Index   293
About the Author   301

LIST OF ILLUSTRATIONS

MAJOR BODY SPLITS

2-1. Right/Left Split   26
2-2. Top/Bottom Split   26
2-3. Front/Back Split   27
2-4. Head/Body Split   27
2-5. Torso/Limbs Split   27
2-6. Small Top, Large Bottom   35
2-7. Large Top, Small Bottom   35
3-1. Healthy Foot, Showing Three Points of Contact
     with the Ground   51
3-2. Healthy, Well-Grounded Foot   52
3-3. Flat Foot   52
3-4. Clutching Foot   54
3-5. Heel-Digging Foot   54
3-6. Foot Reflexology Chart: Right Foot   62
3-7. Foot Reflexology Chart: Left Foot   63
4-1. Pelvis Tipped Upward   82
4-2. Pelvis Tipped Downward   84
4-3. The Seven Kundalini Chakras   88
4-4. First Chakra: The Root Chakra   92
4-5. Anal-Region Holding, Showing Pinching In of
     Buttocks   95

4-6. Anal-Region Holding, Showing Pulling In and Up
  of Pelvic Floor   96

4-7. Second Chakra: The Spleen or Splenic Chakra   99

4-8. Typical Orgasm Cycle in the Male   104

5-1. Third Chakra: The Navel or Umbilical Chakra   121

6-1. Fourth Chakra: The Heart or Cardiac Chakra   149

6-2. Contracted Chest   156

6-3. Expanded Chest   160

7-1. Bowed, Rounded Shoulders   166

7-2. Raised Shoulders   167

7-3. Square Shoulders   169

7-4. Forward, Hunched Shoulders   171

7-5. Retracted, or Pulled-Back, Shoulders   171

8-1. Fifth Chakra: Throat or Laryngeal Chakra   188

8-2. Receding Jaw   200

8-3. Protruding Jaw   202

9-1. Large, Round Eyes   224

9-2. Bulging Eyes   224

9-3. Deep-Set Eyes   225

9-4. "Baby Eyes"   225

9-5. Iris Diagnosis Chart: Right Eye   232

9-6. Iris Diagnosis Chart: Left Eye   233

9-7. Sclera Diagnosis Chart: Right Eye   234

9-8. Sclera Diagnosis Chart: Left Eye   235

9-9. Sixth Chakra: Brow or Frontal Chakra   239

10-1. Seventh Chakra: Crown or Coronal Chakra   257

PREFACE

THIS BOOK GREW out of my need to have a comprehensive system for viewing some of the ways the mind and body interface. In my work as a psychologist and gerontologist, and in my private life, I am persistently confronted with the challenge of understanding how personal growth, character, physical structure, and health/dis-ease relate to one another. Before completing the research out of which this book emerged, I did not feel that there existed a system that could do this in a holistic and clear fashion that would be functional for therapists and lay people alike. In fact, beyond the somatotyping system developed by Sheldon,[1] the kinesic interpretation system devised by Birdwhistell and his colleagues,[2] and the complex therapeutic-analysis systems of Reich[3] and Lowen,[4] there have been no reliably effective means for interrelating these crucially important aspects of our lives. It would even seem that many of our medical, educational, religious, and philosophical institutions base their working philosophies on the assumption that such a system and, indeed, such a set of direct relationships do not even exist.

During the six years I spent researching this book, I set out to explore the bodymind from a variety of perspectives. My intention was to blend my own findings and observations with the discoveries of several of the pioneers in this field, such as Wilhelm Reich, Alexander Lowen, William Schutz, Ida Rolf, Moshe Feldenkrais, Fritz Perls, Stanley Keleman, and Hector Prestera, and with several of the yoga disciplines in order to articulate a definitive yet simple system of bodymind reading and mapping. I wanted this system to be creatively holistic and also unattached to any one therapy process: it had to be a system that would apply to the bodymind in states of health and wellness as well as dis-ease.

In this book, I present the bodymind diagnosis system that evolved out of these years of exploration and study, and I use, as an outline for the discussion, the shape and form of the physical body. I have chosen to offer this material in a personal fashion, for I feel that it becomes most real when it is attached to life.

Although the theories and interpretations in this book suggest a variety of remedial and therapeutic possibilities, I have been careful not to present a panacean therapeutic system or process. I believe that a holistic and growth-oriented therapy/education form demands a more in-depth explication of the human body and psyche than is appropriate here. It is also my belief that before any therapy or growth process truly can work, there must be a state of self-awareness and bodymindfulness. Such is the principal focus of this book.

To keep the emphasis on letting you learn more about yourself, I will present a variety of opportunities for you to explore and examine who and what you are, without my telling you whether you are right or wrong. When I offer case studies and clinical examples, I only do so in order to illustrate more fully the particular bodymind relationships that I am discussing, rather than to demonstrate any individual therapy process in detail.

The bodymind therapies and activities that are presented here were chosen because I have had some degree of personal experience with them, and because I have found that in their form and theory they offer a great deal of worthwhile information about bodymind development. I have inserted these discussions into the overall tapestry of this book at points that I feel are especially appropriate, either because of the theoretical content or because of the relationships that exist between specific techniques and important aspects of my own bodymind development. This should not be misconstrued to mean that each of these techniques is designed for a specific bodymind part. All of the methods and therapies that I have chosen to describe are quite capable of dealing with the entire bodymind. Because of the limits of my own experience and the structure of this book, I have not included a discussion of the work of F. M. Alexander,[5] the Lomi School,[6] psychomotor therapy,[7] the Arica School,[8] dance therapy,[9] and several other important approaches.

I would like to apologize to men and women for my consistent use of the masculine gender for pronouns and collective nouns throughout the book. Because there are no words in the English language that successfully combine third-person genders like he/she and him/her, I have chosen to work within the limits of our language.

Nor does our language support the notion of body/mind unity. As a result, I have had to make use of old as well as several new words in order to express myself most accurately. Throughout this book, I use the word *body* to refer to the purely "physical" aspects of a human being. As long as a person is alive, he is never just a body separated from mind, yet for the purposes of descriptive observation and theoretical discussion, I will use the word in this fashion. I use the word *bodymind* where I wish to refer to both the "physical" *and* the "psychological" aspects of an individual.

K. D.

Berkeley, California
April 1985

ACKNOWLEDGMENTS

I would like to extend my deepest appreciation and love
to . . .

My grandmother, who is perfect

My grandfather, a great man—noble, simple, and loving

Karen Cassel, for her love, support, patience, and soft beauty

Mike Frank, who has always been there for me . . . my best friend

Bill Newman, who took my head and spun it around a few times,
for being such a loving friend

Frank Wuest, whose faith, love, and support have many times
served to keep me upright, for staying close

Will Schutz, who taught me how to "see" and how to "pay attention," two of the most valuable tools I possess, for introduc-
ing me to the "bodymind"

Gay Luce, for being the most "human" being I have ever experienced, a rare woman, and for allowing the love to pass
between us

Jean Houston, who wakes me up when I fall asleep and pokes me
when I get numb

Don Gerrard, who gently guided me to a comfortable style of
writing, for being so supportive and helpful and available
and loving

Eugenia Gerrard, who caught me in midair and eased me gently
to the ground, for inspiring me with her own evolution

Goodwin Watson, who jostled and provoked me into educating myself

Jad King and Juan Barberis, for their masterful artwork

Jana Reiser, for typing and typing and typing and smiling

Joanna Taylor and Ursula Bender, whose editorial comments helped me to crystallize my thoughts

The Esalen Family, who showed me that I could get color from my black-and-white set

. . . and everyone else whom I love and care about. Thank you.

FOREWORD

THIS BOOK IS everything a reader could ask for: a warm, clear, valuable, careful account of a universally relevant topic—the astonishing relationship between body and mind.

Well-being cannot be infused intravenously or ladled out by prescription. Western medicine is beginning to recognize that health and disease don't just happen to us. They are part of a matrix: the bodymind. They are active processes issuing from inner harmony or disharmony, profoundly affected by our states of consciousness, our ability or inability to flow with experience. They reflect psychological and somatic harmony.

As more is learned in brain research, the connection between mind and illness becomes more understandable. The brain masterminds or indirectly influences every function of the body: blood pressure, heart rate, immune responses, hormones, everything. Its mechanisms are linked by an alarm network, and it has a kind of dark genius, organizing disorders appropriate to our most neurotic imaginings.

All illness, whether cancer or schizophrenia or a cold, originates in the bodymind. On his deathbed, Louis Pasteur acknowledged that a medical adversary of his had been right in insisting that disease is caused less by the germ than by the resistance of the individual invaded by the germ. The old saying, "Name your poison," applies to the semantics and symbols of disease. If we feel "picked on," or someone gives us a "pain in the neck," we may make our metaphors literal—with acne or neck spasms. People have long spoken of a "broken heart" as the result of a disappointing relationship; now research shows a connection between loneliness and heart disease. So the broken heart may become coronary disease; ambivalence, a splitting headache; and the rigid personality, arthritis.

Over the years our bodies become walking autobiographies that tell friends and strangers alike of the major and minor stresses of our lives. For instance, distortions of function that occur after an injury—like a limited range of motion in a hurt arm—become a permanent part of our body pattern. Our musculature also reflects old anxieties. Poses of timidity, depression, bravado, or stoicism adopted early in life are locked into our bodies as patterns in our sensorimotor system.

In the vicious cycle of bodymind pathology, our body's tight patterns contribute to our locked-in mental processes. We cannot separate mental from physical, fact from fantasy, past from present. Just as the body feels the mind's grief, so the mind is constricted by the body's stubborn memory of what the mind *used to feel.*

One essential way in which this cycle can be interrupted is through "bodywork"—therapies that deeply (and often painfully) massage, manipulate, loosen, or otherwise change the body's neuromuscular system and its orientation to gravity, its symmetry. Bodywork alters the flow of energy through the body, freeing it of its old "ideas" or patterns, increasing its range of movement. Changing the body in this way can affect the entire bodymind loop.

Drawing on the works of Wilhelm Reich, Ida Rolf, Moshe Feldenkrais, Fritz Perls, William Schutz, Alexander Lowen, and several yoga schools, Ken Dychtwald blends their insights with a variety of Eastern and Western approaches to bodymind development. He peddles no particular school of bodywork or psychotherapy, instead he examinines these theorists with appreciation and synthesis. He has experienced personally a variety of systems, worked with some of these great pioneers, and led his own workshops; it's hard to believe that he wrote this book at the age of twenty-six.

Making a strong case for the shaping of the body by experience, Ken Dychtwald disarmingly uses himself as Exhibit A. There is none of the self-righteousness found in many books on getting your body right. He reassures us by again using himself as an example; "In my own life, I have given up on the notion of the 'perfect' bodymind or the 'ideal life,' for there is no such thing."

The author takes the reader on a journey that lets us discover the bodymind connection together. Traveling, chapter by chapter, through the physical shape and form of the body, blending contemporary theories, firsthand experience, and ancient wisdom, he helps us see that the body not only reflects all the historical and present conflicts of the mind, but that the reorganization of one helps reorganize the other. This recognition carries with it implicit responsibility and opportunity. Recognizing this, Ken Dychtwald takes us that extra step, which allows us to explore the various ways we can intervene in our own bodymind loop so that we can take steps toward self-responsibility in the pursuit of our own health and well-being.

Prepare yourself for an adventure into yourself exploring the astonishing relationship between psyche and soma.

Marilyn Ferguson

BODYMIND

CHAPTER

1

BODY/MIND

IT IS SEPTEMBER 1970. I am standing naked before a roomful of men and women of all ages. Dr. John Pierrakos is staring intently at my body, as are all the other people in the room. The heat from their stares is combining with the warmth of the Southern California air to make me a little light in the head and shaky on my legs. Yet I continue to stand and be observed.

Dr. Pierrakos walks toward me and carefully examines the texture of my skin and the overall quality of my body's musculature. He asks me to walk around the room for a few moments so that he can observe my body in motion. As I walk, I am aware of my own self-consciousness and awkwardness. Being observed and scrutinized so intently by a group of people is an activity I am not very good at. The butterflies in my stomach are beginning to flap and screech as I return to my waiting position in front of the room. I am sweating profusely from the intensity of the situation.

After what seems like seven hitless innings of silence, John Pierrakos proceeds to tell me about myself with a voice that is simultaneously whimsical and stern. For me,

there are no other sounds in the universe. I listen carefully.
He tells me about my mother and my father and about my
relationship to both of them. He describes my general attitudes regarding life, love, relationships, movement,
change, and performance. With remarkable accuracy, he
discusses the sorts of relationships and styles of behavior
that I would naturally seek out and tells me about the way
I deal with them. For a finale, he describes my major personality strengths and weaknesses. As he talks, the other
people in the room listen carefully. Some of them are busy
jotting down notes, others are nodding their heads in ap-
proval, and others have eyes closed as if to scrutinize some
internal picture. John Pierrakos finishes staring at me.

What was frightening about this experience was that everything he said, every observation he made, every description he offered, was entirely accurate. He concisely described me to me. How did he do it? How could he possibly
know so much about my feelings and my life? We had just
met the day before and I had revealed none of my personal
life to him.

I sat down and drifted in and out of deep thought as one
after another of the members of the group stood up to be
scrutinized by John Pierrakos. And one after another, each
of them nodded their heads in confirmation as he accurately introduced each of them to themselves. There was an
obvious certainty to his perceptions that suggested real
awareness of who and what each of us was. But there
seemed to be no way that he could have known about our
minds and personalities by just looking at our bodies. His
ability to understand immediately our basic natures suggested that there must have been some source from which
he found out all this information.

The question was: Who would be so totally and intimately aware of each of our lives? What source would know
so well how we molded and created our selves? The more
I questioned, the more confused I seemed to get, until

finally I realized who and what my informer was. It was my *body*—the body that I had taken with me to the workshop, the body that had been with me since birth, the body that I had trained and nurtured throughout my life. Somehow, this body, my body, was presenting information about me to John Pierrakos that he was noticing and reading back to me.

How could this possibly be? How could my body be so expressive of my inner self? How could my life history be seen in the way my muscles were shaped? If I was my body, then who was responsible for its, my, well-being and health? Did my body shape my mind or did my mind shape my body? If I had had a hand in forming myself, then how responsible was I for all my creations and actions, health and dis-ease? Questions poured out of me by the dozens. The implications of these questions and their possible answers not only suggested a greater appreciation of my own personal self-responsibility but also demanded a revaluation of all my beliefs and attitudes concerning nearly everything pertaining to my personal health and well-being. It forced me to reconsider every aspect of my life and beingness. But before I tell you more about my growing recognition of psychosomatic unity, let me first share with you an image of what it was like when I still "had" a body.

In those days, my body was with me always. It walked with me, ran with me, slept with me, laughed with me, and followed me wherever I went. I spent a fair amount of time grooming my body, training it to perform and present itself in ways that were appropriate to my needs. I taught my body how to play tennis, how to look attractive, how to make love, how to behave, and most important, I taught it how to obey me.

Over the years, my body and I shared many wonderful experiences and stimulating encounters. Because of the nature of our relationship we were forced to participate in

each other's interests and activities. For example, when I
went off to college, my body, of course, came with me. In
class, my body would have to sit patiently while I was being
educated. This education didn't include my body, so it
would have to wait till after class, when I would take it to
the gym and let it run around to work off the tension it had
developed while waiting for me in class.

I especially appreciated my body when it served me well
and when it allowed me to feel that I was healthy and alive.
I dreaded the time when my body would begin to deterio-
rate. I had seen this happen to other bodies and had noticed the way the people inside these bodies reacted to
these imperfections. It was my hope that my body would
remain attractive and functional as long as I needed its
services. I felt that if I kept it well fed and well tuned, then
the least it could do would be to show its appreciation to
me by maintaining its responsiveness and servility.

Usually, my body responded in a respectable manner,
but sometimes I would lose control of it, and it would twist
or break or carry on in ways that were definitely not very
becoming. During those periods of injury and dis-ease I
was angry and impatient with my body. I was annoyed that
it had gotten sick and by so doing had temporarily ruined
my life. I was also always impatient with it for not healing
up very quickly, or at least not as quickly as I would have
liked. In order to speed up its healing I would fill it up with
chemicals that were meant to remedy whatever problems
were ailing it. I'm not sure if my body liked these chemicals
or not, but that wasn't important because they usually
seemed to work, and after a little while, my body would be
up and about again. During these times of stress and sickness I was always confronted with how very little I knew
about my body. Even though we had lived together for so
long, I was still ignorant about how it functioned and generated itself.

When these times of bodily breakdown occurred, I would

usually blame my body for its inadequacies. Sometimes I even blamed my parents' bodies, for it was from their bodies that mine had been created. I believed that my body was simply living out its genetic code, and therefore, when it malfunctioned, it was obviously because of the inadequacies in my parents' bodies, passed on to me.

There were also times when I abused my body. That is, there were occasions when I didn't feed it properly or give it enough rest or give it the exercise and oxygen that it needed. During those times, however, I was convinced that I was involved in more important matters; my body could wait.

I also found that I could totally ignore my body for long stretches of time and, except for helping out with necessary biological functions, could separate myself from it completely. During those times I would continue living my life, and as long as my body could maintain its health, we would have no conflict. However, my body always needed some attention from me in order to survive, my body was totally dependent on me. I was the brains behind both of us, and my body would never let me forget how childlike and demanding it was with its wild actions, desires, and needs. Even though my body was considered attractive and well functioning, I often found myself resenting it for demanding so much from me without giving very much in return.

There were other times, however, when my body brought me great pleasure and satisfaction. Because of its neuromuscular apparatus, my body had the potential for pleasure and vitality as well as pain and sickness. Sometimes, with my permission, it would engage in activities such as lovemaking or sports or relaxation that brought me pleasure and an accompanying release from life's tensions. These experiences were highly enjoyable, and during these moments my body and I became close friends.

After coexisting for twenty years with my body in this symbiotic fashion, I happened to bring it with me to a variety of growth centers and educational facilities in California, where I was studying different aspects of the human potential movement. I had expected to engage in these experiences and studies without the involvement of my body, but I soon discovered that my body and I were related in an entirely different fashion than I had previously come to believe. The experience with John Pierrakos proved to be the first of a long series of experiences and realizations that served to reshape totally the relationship I was having with my body . . . with my self. It was at this time that I stopped "having" a body and first began to realize that I "am" my body and that my body "is" *me.*

So now I was forced to confront the possibility that my body was revealing through its form and flows my story, my history, my life. Apparently each curve and muscle told of a certain chapter and a certain constellation of relationships, the accumulation of which had become my self-image, had become "me." John Pierrakos is one of the people who knows how to read these forms, how to translate these flows, and how to interpret these stories. He was simply translating me back to me. Apparently, I had translated me into flesh each time I created or re-created myself, and he was simply translating this flesh back into the stories, experiences, and feelings that had shaped the flesh. He was reading my life from my body as an archaeologist might read Egyptian history from its hieroglyphics.

The potential implications of this experience shook me at my roots. The realization that I could be seen from the outside as accurately or perhaps more accurately than I was seeing myself from the inside simply would not fit into anything that I had come to believe about my mind or my body. Everything that I had come to know about my body and my mind and about sickness and health relied upon the belief that I was only partially related to my body, that my body and mind, while stuck together, were not responsible for each other.

This experience took place at a growth center called Kairos, in Rancho Santa Fe, California. The workshop was being led by drs. Alexander Lowen, John Pierrakos, and Stanley Keleman and was focused on a therapeutic process called "bioenergetics." There were fifty people in the workshop, many of whom were well-known bioenergetic therapists.

Bioenergetics is a form of psychotherapy that deals with emotional health and sickness from the perspective of psychosomatic unity and has made enormous contributions to the clinical understanding of the relationships between character and physical structure. Bioenergetic theory and practice are an offspring of the work and beliefs of the late Wilhelm Reich (who will be discussed in greater detail in Chapter 4), one of the early pioneers in the use of therapeutic processes that treat not only mental and emotional symptoms and disorders but their somatic (body) counterparts as well. The bioenergetic process was originally conceived and developed by two of Reich's students, drs. Alexander Lowen and John Pierrakos, in the late 1950s, as an attempt to create a contemporary therapeutic process that effectively combined verbal/intellectual, physical, and psychoemotional means for exploring and resolving body-mind conflict.[1]

The body-reading process that I experienced with Dr. Pierrakos is explained by Alexander Lowen in the following passage:

The character of the individual as it is manifested in his typical pattern of behavior is also portrayed on the somatic level by the form and movement of the body. The sum total of the muscular tensions seen as a gestalt . . . constitutes the "body expression" of the organism. The body expression is the somatic view of the typical emotional expression which is seen on the psychic level as "character."[2]

Within the bioenergetic framework there are a variety of "characters" and "body expressions" that are identified as being unhealthy and neurotic. By carefully diagnosing the physical and psychological condition of his patient, the bioenergetic therapist hopes to arrive at a more complete understanding of the way in which this individual has come to shape his life and himself. Once the therapist has completed his diagnosis, he proceeds to work with the patient with a variety of carefully developed verbal, psychoemotional, and physical activities and exercises that are designed to unblock the areas of tension, strengthen the points of vitality, and encourage the sources of personal growth and, thereby, dissolve the unhealthy behavior.

Before this workshop, I had heard a lot of discussion about mind-body relationships, but nearly all these discussions were intellectually oriented and abstract. My introduction to bioenergetics was my first direct experience with being forced to encounter myself as a psychosomatic unity in a way that I simply could not discount.

It is November 1970. I am attending my first workshop at Esalen Institute in Big Sur, California. At the time, Esalen has been well known for a few years as an outrageous, avantgarde center for the exploration of "those trends in education, religion, philosophy, and the physical and behavioral sciences which emphasize the potentialities and values of human existence."[3] The institute draws some of its colorful dynamics from its location amidst the violently peaceful cliffs and woods of the Big Sur coastline just south of Carmel, California.

The workshop is being led by drs. Hector Prestera and William Schutz. I have been enticed to sign up for this workshop by curiosity about Dr. Schutz, who developed the highly controversial "open encounter" process,[4] and because I am fascinated with the title of the workshop: "Bodymind." I have never seen that word before, and it suggests to me a recognition of the holistic interrelationship of body and mind. I am hoping that this workshop will help to enlighten me a bit more about these relationships and will also allow me to learn more about my own newly discovered "bodymind."

In this workshop, which is to run for seven days with nine hours of meetings per day, Schutz and Prestera have decided to combine encounter with Rolfing. What this means is that in addition to the usual encounter therapy, concentrating on interpersonal sharing and exploring, special time will be devoted to exploring the ways by which each of us shapes and structures his own body, ways that perhaps relate to our unique characters.[5]

Rolfing, or "structural integration," as it is officially called, is a system of deep muscular manipulation and massage that has been developed by a biochemist and physiologist named Ida Rolf. During the many years that she has been examining muscle tissue and cell structure Dr. Rolf has come to notice that physical and emotional traumas seem to tighten and rigidify the muscular and fascial tissues of the body. When this happens, the body tends to move out of a state of natural alignment and vitality and into a condition of overall inflexibility and gravitational imbalance. In addition, the continual rigidification of the body also serves to limit the range of emotional flexibility of which the unrestricted body is capable. This point is clearly made in the following passage by Ida Rolf:

An individual experiencing temporary fear, grief, or anger, all too often carries his body in an attitude which the world recognizes as the outward manifestation of that particular emotion. If he persists in this dramatization or consistently re-establishes it, thus forming what is ordinarily referred to as a "habit pattern," the muscular arrangement becomes set.

Materially speaking, some muscles shorten and thicken, others are invaded by connective tissue, still others become immobilized by consolidation of the tissue involved. Once this has happened, the physical attitude is invariable; it is involuntary; it can no longer be changed basically by taking thought or even by mental suggestion. Such setting of a physical response also establishes an emotional pattern. Since it is not possible to establish a free flow through the physical flesh, the subjective emotional tone becomes progressively more limited and tends to remain in a restricted, closely defined area. Now what the individual feels is no longer an emotion, a response to an immediate situation, henceforth he lives, moves and has his being in an attitude.[6]

In response to this bodymind dilemma, Dr. Rolf has devised a system of ten therapeutic sessions that are aimed at allowing the body to assume a more healthy and integrated position with respect to itself and the continual pull of gravity.[7] In the Rolfing process, the trained practitioner deeply massages the body in order to free up muscles and fasciae and to allow the body to assume a more fully integrated posture. By releasing the chronically held traumas of a lifetime and reconnecting the natural flows and balances of the organism, the Rolf system seeks to increase health and vitality, to alleviate stress and tension, and to encourage growth and openness on all levels of organismic functioning. Because the massage work is deep, the Rolfee may also experience some emotional and energetic release during the process.

Both Schutz and Prestera are trained Rolf practitioners; they are professionals in other areas as well—the first a psychotherapist, the latter a practicing internist. This workshop was one of the first times that two great therapists from diverse backgrounds joined together to pool skills and talents regarding bodymind awareness and growth in an experimental clinical setting.

On the second day of the workshop, there are twelve of us sitting in a circle around one of the group members, who is being Rolfed simultaneously by Schutz and Prestera. The Rolfee is being encouraged to express himself and his emotions in any way that he wishes during the Rolfing experience.

As the Rolfers' hands move over and into the body, the subject responds with sadness, fear, joy, and memories that seem to come up from nowhere. Schutz and Prestera are being very careful to take the time and patience to allow the Rolfee an opportunity to work through the emotional content of the information that is emerging during the deep massage work.

As the days pass and our group grows closer, and trust and caring develop, we begin to feel each other's pains and pleasures with a great deal of openness and sensitivity. It is interesting to me to note that each of us responds to certain aspects of another's ordeal and that each of our reactions seems to be unique to our own natures. I am reminded of the first time I learned to tune a guitar. I was amazed to find that when I struck a particular note on one string, the same note resonated on the other strings. In very much the same way, it seems that each of us is tuned to a variety of notes and chords (feelings and attitudes), and when these sounds or feelings are struck in our presence, the natural response is to resonate.

Each day two more of us are Rolfed as part of the group process, and each day I watch as each Rolfee responds to the Rolfing in a slightly different fashion. Since the "number one" Rolfing session—the one being practiced here— is a standard procedure, most variation in response is due to individual experience rather than to variations in pressure or movement on the part of the Rolfer.

As I watch more and more people being Rolfed and sharing their emotions and fantasies with the group, I begin to notice that many similar stories are being recalled and abreacted by different members of the group. What is stranger is that these *similar* stories come up when *similar* parts of *different* Rolfees' bodies are confronted.

For example, feelings and memories of being left and neglected repeatedly appear when a Rolfee's chest is being released. When the upper back is worked on, the muscular confrontation is often accompanied by strong feelings of rage and anger. Rolfed jaws release sadness; Rolfed hips release sexuality; Rolfed shoulders seem invariably to tell stories of burdens and stressful responsibilities. It appears that the body is like a large circuit board: when certain neuromuscular switches are contacted and opened, similar stories and experiences emerge from the same body parts belonging to different people.

At first, this does not seem possible. I am having a hard enough time buying the notion that emotions are stored in the body, let alone believing that there is a general order by which they store themselves. Yet, as each day passes and I watch more and more bodies being freed, this possibility seems less and less unreasonable. I become fascinated with the idea that the body is a storehouse for emotions and beliefs. I watch as people walk, as they talk, as they emote, and as they move.

By apprenticing myself to Schutz and Prestera, I got to watch them Rolf nearly one hundred different people during the next four months. At the same time I participated in an encounter therapy training program for over one thousand intense hours. This allowed me to observe intimately hundreds of nude bodies in the process of interacting and emoting. During these months the workshop room became a living laboratory for me, in which I would watch the bodymind in action. With a passion that verged on fanaticism, I made mental notes to myself about what sorts of people were shaped in what sorts of ways. Conversely, I examined bodies and tried to imagine what sorts of people and personalities they housed and reflected. I would look at the physical structure of those who were being Rolfed and try to guess the ways in which they would relate to the contact of Rolfing and to imagine the sort of memories and blocks that would be released by the Rolfing experience.

As the months passed, I found that my feelings and observations were leading me to develop a philosophical system that accounted for the direct relationships between particular feelings and beliefs and specific body parts and regions. It was during this time that I began to work through the confusion that my initial encounter with John Pierrakos had created. I began to learn how to translate the mind into the body and the body back into the mind. It was also during these months that I began to cultivate the conceptual framework that I am presenting to you in this book.

In the six years between that time and the completion of this book I continued to delve deeper and deeper into the questions and practices that probe the relationships between body and mind, health and dis-ease. During these years I have also continued to develop and refine a comprehensive system of bodymind reading and mapping that allows one to read the personality from the flows and form of the body and to understand the psychosomatic nature of health and dis-ease. By immersing myself personally and professionally in the fields of human-potential exploration and personal growth, my studies and explorations have led me through many bodymind techniques, such as Rolfing, bioenergetics, Reichian energetics, encounter therapy, massage, Shiatsu, healing, the Feldenkrais method, Gestalt therapy, and a variety of yoga practices. In addition, I have examined related areas such as biofeedback, meditation, psychodrama, sensory awareness, psychedelicism, and an exploration of the nature of the psychotic experience.

I have been exploring from a variety of perspectives and through a variety of styles what it is, and what it might be, to be a human being in this world. In essence, I have been trying to organize information and experience in such a way as to allow for the creation of an alternative mythology of human be-ing, based on the sorts of recognitions and relationships that I, and an expanding number of other people, have been discovering and exploring. The priorities that result from these discoveries have to do with increased awareness, larger self-responsibility, enhanced health, and an overall appreciation of the forces of life/ death that are continually at play within each of us.

My focus has been on the heightening of the quality of life and on discovering the beliefs and practices that lend themselves to the enhancement of this goal. My working assumptions have been that we can all be a bit more alive and human, and that there are a variety of practices and attitudes that lend themselves to this end.

In this book, I would like to share with you some of the beliefs and experiences that have fascinated and guided me in this regard. I shall focus my discussion on the nature of the human bodymind. While I surely will not be able to communicate all my feelings and beliefs regarding the ways in which the bodymind comes to be, I will attempt to share and explore some of my observations and experiences regarding several of the most basic bodymind relationships and related therapeutic activities.

This book is a blend of psychosomatic theory, diagnostic descriptions and illustrations, and personal reflections all contained within practical discussions of ways to experience, explore, and expand the limits of human be-ing. The outline I will be using for my discussion is that of the human body, for I have discovered that not only is it the most vital and exciting of all energetic forms, but it also provides the perfect structure through which to generate an exploration of bodymind unity, health, and creative self-development.

After I have discussed some of the basic qualities and

characteristics of the bodymind in the next chapter, I will proceed to work my way upward from the feet to the top of the head, examining, describing, and exploring many of the more specific bodymind parts and relationships.[8] In addition, I have chosen to present some of my own experiences and reflections regarding my own bodymind and several of the most popular bodymind techniques, not within a separate chapter but, instead, at appropriate locations throughout this bodymind journey.

CHAPTER

OVERVIEW

IF YOU WERE to take a close look at me, you might comment
on how healthy and well-proportioned I am. If you were a
physician, you would probably say that I am in good health
and that I am lucky to have such a vital, well-toned body.
When I examine myself closely, however, I notice that there
are all sorts of imbalances, confusions, and rough edges
alive within my tissue as surely as they are alive within my
soul, conflicts that have come to form my physical body as
definitely and as distinctly as they have also served to mold
my character and life.

In fact, my body is incredibly lopsided. My right leg is
longer than my left; my left hand is smaller than my right;
my right shoulder is lower than my left; the top half of my
body is more muscular than the bottom half; my pelvis is
rotated a bit in a clockwise fashion; my neck is angled
slightly to the right; my spine is not as straight as it is
supposed to be; my feet are somewhat archless; my right
hand is more coordinated than my left hand; my left leg is
tighter than my right leg . . . and on and on. There is an

infinity of asymmetries and imbalances within my body.

I am not smooth, for my life has not always been smooth. I am not perfectly balanced, for my feelings are not always balanced. I am not symmetrical, for my actions are not symmetrical. My muscular strength is not equally proportioned throughout my body, as my interests are not equally distributed throughout my life. In a way, my body is like the body of the earth, which with its mountains, valleys, riverbeds, and uneven topography tells the story of its history and creation as surely as my body expresses the trials and creative changes that I have experienced throughout my lifetime. Every aspect of my body reflects a distinct aspect of my self, which, extending outward from my psyche and embodied in flesh, encounters the passions and challenges with which I am continually engaged.

In my attempt to explore the terrain of my own life and being, I have discovered that my body and my mind are reflections of each other and that the emotions and experiences which have formed my personality have affected the formation and structuring of my muscles and tissue. As I have become more aware of my own history and the realm of possibilities that it reveals, I have also come to appreciate some of the ways that these body/mind relationships can be discovered, examined, and improved upon.

As we explore the different aspects of the bodymind and examine how these areas of life are embodied within us, please do not use this information as another way to be critical of yourself but rather as a way to appreciate your own specialness. As you learn to read your own bodymind, allow yourself to enjoy the way your muscles and limbs have come to tell the stories that are alive within you, stories that tell of experiences past, passions present, and dreams future. By becoming more aware of the distinctions within your own bodymind, you will find yourself empowered with greater self-awareness.

In my own life, I have given up on the notion of the

"perfect" bodymind or the "ideal" life, for there are no such things. Rather, I have been allowing myself to become more aware and enlightened about my own potentialities and by so doing have begun to discover the unique life and bodymind that is "ideal" for my specific needs and dreams. I notice that when I approach my growth and self-explorations from this perspective, they become pleasurable adventures rather than tedious chores.[1]

FORMATION OF THE BODYMIND

Traditionally, five components have been identified as influential in the formation of the human bodymind: (1) heredity, (2) physical activity and exposure, (3) emotional and psychological activity and exposure, (4) nutrition, and (5) environment.

Heredity includes all those factors that are with us at birth. This information and structure is passed on from our parents to us and is, no doubt, a critical factor in the formation of our own unique bodyminds. For obvious reasons, it is very difficult to isolate those aspects of the physical and psychological self for which heredity is entirely responsible.

The second influential component, *physical activity*, includes all the physical actions, activities, and encounters that we experience throughout our lives. Walking, sleeping, bicycle riding, exercising, pounding nails, sitting, giving birth, and playing the piano are all activities that, regardless of their hereditary and psychoemotional components, serve to mold and shape our bodyminds. What we have done with our selves, how we have done it, how frequently we have done it, and how it felt to be doing it are all reflected in the way we have developed our muscles, bones, and neuromuscular coordination.

While it is often the physical activity with which we involve ourselves that allows us to grow and develop in a healthy, vital fashion, sometimes physical activity can also be responsible for limitations in optimal bodymind development. This possibility is well exemplified by William Schutz in the following statement:

> Physical trauma can interfere with my natural growth process . . . just as pruning reduces a full grown tree to a midget bonsai. Suppose I break an ankle early in my life. During the healing process, I feel unsteady on my feet and throw my weight forward on my toes. If I do not compensate for this imbalance, I will fall forward. I may compensate by tightening the muscles in the small of my back. If these muscles become too strong, I will fall backward: thus, I must make another compensation by thrusting my head forward. When I balance my body in this way, the muscles in my legs, back and neck feel tense.
>
> If I adopt this posture, eventually the muscle tensions become chronic, and my connective tissue grows to hold these muscles in a rigid position. My muscles lose their ability to flex and relax appropriately.[2]

The third component, *emotional and psychological activity and exposure,* is the one that fascinates me the most. While most people will agree that feelings, attitudes, and experiences have an effect on the conditions of their bodymind, there is very little agreement about *how much* effect they have. For example, if I am nervous and I feel butterflies in my stomach, I naturally relate my physical symptoms to the emotional stress. Or, if I have just had a fight with my girlfriend and I notice that my neck is stiff and I've got a headache coming on, I'll probably admit to myself that the argument caused the tension.

Yet, how far will I carry these psychosomatic associations? When I have a sore throat, do I associate it with restrained anger? If I sprain my ankle, did I do so at a time when I was feeling emotionally ungrounded? If I am asthmatic, am I this way because it is hard for me to take responsibility for the rage that is trapped in my chest? If I have

hemorrhoids, is it because I have been holding on to all of
my feelings too tightly? If I am blissfully happy, is it because
my bodymind is healthfully relaxed and integrated?

Chances are that most of us do not relate all our emotional attitudes and experiences to specific physical symptoms and conditions. Conversely, how many of us translate
our body structure into personality preferences and emotional history? Yet, there is increasing evidence that our
feelings and attitudes very directly affect the way we hold
ourselves, move, breathe, and grow, and that just as we
partly form ourselves with physical activity, so do we mold
ourselves with selective emotional activity and experience.

For example, imagine that you are extremely nervous
and upset. With this feeling, allow the accompanying physical sensations in your belly and, perhaps, a shortening of
breath. What would happen if you practiced this psychosomatic pattern for a few minutes each day? Surely after
months and years of exercising yourself in this fashion, the
muscles of your belly and chest would begin to shape themselves in reflection of this state of nervousness with its
accompanying tensions and blockages.

Or imagine that you are very unhappy and depressed.
Allow yourself to assume the posture that would embody
these feelings. Chances are, your shoulders would slump,
your chest would become sunken in, and you would project
an overall feeling of heaviness.

Emotional stimulation of muscles can have the same
effect on the body as purely physical activity, except that it
is usually more difficult to detect the source of stimulation
and the way in which it has been selectively, and often
unconsciously, exercised. The body begins to form around
the feelings that animate it, and the feelings, in turn, become habituated and trapped within the body tissue itself.
The bodymind then, when seen from this perspective, is to
some extent the continually regenerating product of a lifetime of emotional encounters, psychological activities, and
psychosomatic preferences.

The fourth major component in the creation of the body-mind is *nutrition*. By nutrition, I mean all the fuel, psychological as well as physical, that the bodymind takes in and digests in order to supply itself with the necessary elements for regeneration and continued growth.[3] While there is disagreement about what fuels are most healthful or appropriate, there is definite agreement about the important role that nutrition plays in the creation and maintenance of the bodymind.

Environment is the last major component that is influential in the formation of the human bodymind. By environment I mean all the physical, social, and psychological structures within which we live our lives. Like heredity, environmental factors are givens that we receive as we enter into life at a particular time and in a particular location, but they differ from heredity in that we have the ability to change them and, therefore, their influence on our personal development by taking steps to alter them or else by simply changing locations. As a result, our relationship to our environment is a dynamic process that is continually open to change, rearrangement, and re-creation. It is extremely difficult to separate ourselves from our environment, for, in a sense, it lives as much within us as it does outside us.[4]

I have isolated these five approaches for academic purposes, but in reality they are inseparable. In this book, I will focus primarily on the third component of bodymind formation, that of emotional activity and psychological preference. While this path is intimately connected to all the others, I feel that it is the most important in its effect on the ongoing development of the human bodymind. I have come to see that emotional experiences, psychological choices, and personal attitudes and images not only affect the functioning of the human organism but also strongly influence the ways it is shaped and structured. This is not to say that heredity, physical activity, nutrition, and environment do not influence the bodymind; they unquestiona-

bly do. Rather, I am suggesting that when all these forces
are merged in the creation of a human being, the force of
the aware human psyche seems to be the most formatively
powerful of all.

When we try to gain information about the way emotional experiences and expressions are related to physical
structure, another difficulty arises. It is the age-old question of which came first: the chicken or the egg. Do emotional experiences and psychological beliefs shape body
tissue and structure, or does the structure of the body
predispose it to specific emotions and attitudinal sets? The
answer seems to be . . . *both.* Translation from mind to
matter and from matter to mind appears to be a kind of
circular feedback system, with each bit of information and
experience feeding back through tissue and then becoming
information and experience once again.[5] So in trying to
decipher the language of the body or the structure or the
psyche, all we can do is to bring these relationships into
awareness and to recognize that at times the chicken and
the egg cannot be separated at all.

The study of the relationships that exist between the
mind and the body is not new. As long as man has reflected
on his health, his survival, his passions, his thoughts, his
dreams, his life, and his "self," there have been questions
about the nature of this most precious and elusive of all
unknown territories. In the East, as exemplified in the Oriental and Indian cultures, the body and the mind have
traditionally been viewed as inseparable aspects of the
same human essence. The health practices, educational
forms, religious institutions, and psychoemotional disciplines of this part of the planet all suggest a holistic approach to life and self-development. By exploring and developing himself, an individual can achieve harmony within
his bodymind and thereby attain a state of happiness and
bliss.

Here in the West, we have chosen to make a duality of

the bodymind, separating it into two parts: the psyche, which is considered to live somewhere in the skull between the eyes; and the body, which lives and moves beneath it. This mind/body dualism is reflected in all our institutions and cultural processes. By intellectually dividing ourselves into parts, we encourage intensive specialization and differentiation in all our activities, thereby further encouraging mind/body separatism rather than holism. Because of this split, it is not surprising to find that our minds and bodies often compete and argue, for they lack integration.[6]

In the chapters to follow, I will be discussing and describing many different parts of the bodymind. I will be isolating arms, knees, thoughts, and feelings in order to illustrate some of the ways by which we create ourselves in our own image. I will be separating the bodymind, for the purpose of this book, with words, theories, and stories. I must remind you, however, that my purpose in separating the bodymind is to allow you to learn more about the ways that it (you) are not separate at all.

In reality, every cell in your body is both structurally and functionally related to every other cell in your body. Similarly, all your thoughts, beliefs, fears, and dreams are dynamically connected within the structure and function of your psyche. I would also like to suggest that your cells and your thoughts are more directly interconnected than you probably believe at present.

As you experience and study the various bodymind parts and processes that I will be isolating and discussing, please be continually aware that each and every aspect of you is attached and related in some remarkable way to every other aspect of you. By discovering and integrating these relationships, you allow yourself to bring greater harmony into your bodymind, thereby diminishing the conflicts that live within you and increasing your overall health and psychological well-being. Most important, as you journey through yourself, with this book serving as a kind of psychosomatic travelogue, please remember to appreciate your bodymind for its holistic nature, and do not get sidetracked by the theoretical separations and distinctions that will be made.

MAJOR BODYMIND SPLITS

Before I discuss a variety of specifically located psychosomatic relationships, I will first present an analysis of several of the major splits that can be observed in the bodymind, which will allow you to begin to see some of the ways in

**MAJOR BODY
SPLITS**

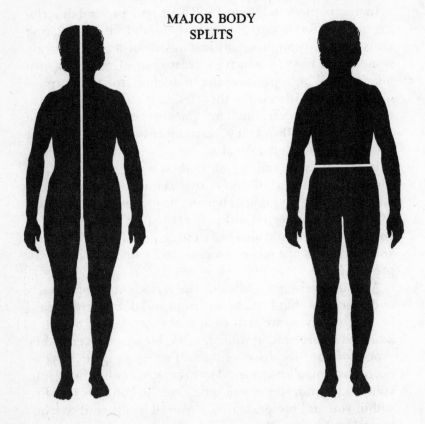

2-1. Right/Left Split   *2-2. Top/Bottom Split*

2-3. *Front/Back Split*

2-4. *Head/Body Split*

2-5. *Torso/Limbs Split*

which the shape of the physical body is reflective of the psychological body that is housed within it. These splits are: right/left, top/bottom, front/back, head/body, torso/limbs.

First, it might be helpful for you to take a few minutes to explore the overall form of your own bodymind. This is best done in the nude, and it is helpful to stand in front of a full-length mirror in order to get a total view of the way your body is shaped.

As you look at yourself, try to be nonjudgmental and avoid commenting to yourself about things you need to be doing for yourself (like dieting or exercising) or changes that have affected your posture (like aging or illness). Simply view yourself and allow yourself to get a sense of the way you are shaped and molded in every part of your body. Pay particular attention to the relationship that exists between the left and right sides of your body. Does one side appear to be larger or more powerful than the other? Is one side more healthy looking than the other?

How about the top and bottom halves of your body? Do they seem to be proportionately related, or is one of the halves larger and heavier than the other? Take a few moments to explore your body with respect to areas of strength or weakness. As you look at yourself, see if you can make a mental map of your body's topography, charting points of vitality and health, as well as points of dis-ease and illness.

Sometimes, it's helpful to make a sketch of your body, front and back, and then color in the various experiences, incidents, and traumas that have contributed to your physical structure. To do this, take a large sheet of paper (perhaps butcher paper) and first outline your body. Then with different colored crayons or pencils draw in all the locations in your body where you have experienced either pain, stress, accident, or illness. Be sure to include all the little injuries and strains as well as the larger dis-eases and problems. Then, with other colors, highlight all the parts of your body that give you, or have given you, great joy or pleasure. Be sure to include all those parts that you consider vital and healthy. You might even discover that some of these locations coincide with the unhealthy zones. When you have completed this part of the drawing, look at yourself and try to get a sense of what parts of your body seem to project a glow of vitality outward to other people. For example, you might feel that your face gives off a pleasant shine, or perhaps your hands generate a great deal of love or energy. In any case, once you have decided what part or parts of you are exceptionally vital and outpouring, color them in on your drawing as auras projecting outward from the surface of your body.

While you are creating this body map, it is important that you take the time to sense how you feel about the different aspects of your body. See if you feel intimate with certain parts of yourself, more of a stranger to other parts. Make notes to yourself about your discoveries and save your drawings (front and back), for these will be helpful as references as we discuss the various bodymind functions and qualities.[7]

Right/Left Split

The first separation that I will deal with is the one that exists between the right and left sides of the bodymind. These sides, while they seem extremely similar to one another, often house and animate different aspects of character and personality. It may be helpful to remember that the left cerebral hemisphere controls most of the right side's motor and neuromuscular functioning, and that the right cerebral hemisphere controls the left side of the body.

In recent years, several fascinating studies have explored right/left brain activity, and these have indicated strong differentiations between the character and quality of right

and left hemisphere activity. According to Dr. Robert Ornstein, a pioneer in this field, the left hemisphere "is
predominantly involved with analytic, logical thinking, especially in verbal and mathematical functions." The right
hemisphere, on the other hand, "is primarily responsible
for orientation in space, artistic endeavors, crafts, body
images, recognition of faces."[8]

Correspondingly, the right side of the bodymind is usually considered the "masculine"[9] side, and as having to do
with logic and rational thought and with such aspects of
personality as assertiveness, aggressiveness, and au-
thoritarianism—in the Chinese cosmology, the yang, or
creative, forces. The left side of the bodymind is considered to be related to the feminine aspects of the character.
Personality constructs such as emotionality, passivity, creative thought, holistic expression, and the yin, or receptive,
forces are said to inhabit and animate this side of the bodymind.

The easiest way to detect the right/left differences is
simply to observe people while they are expressing themselves. The most obvious displays of right/left preferences
occur when emotions are being released and acted out. I
have found that encounter groups, sensitivity workshops,
and group-therapy sessions have proved to be the most
rewarding of all laboratories within which to explore these
psychosomatic relationships.

For example, in December 1970, I participated in an
encounter workshop at Esalen Institute together with
fifteen people of all sizes, shapes, and ages. On the fourth
day of the week-long workshop, we gathered for an afternoon session. The room was bare except for a lushly car-
peted floor and a dozen or so large stuffed pillows that were
on hand for leaning against, sitting on, talking to, kicking,
biting, punching, or just staring at if the session grew dull.

At the time of this particular workshop session, I had
been in encounter therapy training groups continually for

nearly four months, and I was slowly growing bored with the apparent redundancy of people's problems. For diversion, I searched for some new aspect of the encounter situation to focus on. I decided to pay attention to different crying styles, as there always seemed to be quite a bit of crying going on in the groups at Esalen. I didn't have to wait very long. The woman sitting across the room from me, who had been ranting about her husband since the workshop began, unknowingly offered to be the first subject in what must surely have been the first Esalen unofficial "crying" study.

Now that I had a new focus of exploration, I sat up and positioned myself directly across the room from the woman and watched her very carefully as she gestured and expressed her feelings. As she screamed and yelled, I immediately noticed something very strange. It seemed that her tears of rage were flowing almost entirely from her right eye. Assuming that she must have something wrong with the tear ducts in her left eye, I chided myself for having chosen a defective subject on my very first "crying study" case. After a short while of screaming, she began to grow very sad. As she did, the style and rhythm of her crying also changed, from that of anger to that of sadness. What happened next totally surprised me. When her crying and emotions changed from hard to soft, the principal tear source shifted from her right to her left eye. It was as though the tears from her right eye were specifically expressive of hard angry feelings, while her left eye was a tear channel for soft and vulnerable feelings.

Before that instant it had never occurred to me that different types of crying might be related to specific sides of the body. Since that day, I have seen this same right/left crying phenomenon happen many times.

A parallel right/left split is exemplified in the following story that William Schutz relates about an incident that occurred while he was Rolfing a young woman:

As I worked on her right side, I found the tissue tough; her right shoulder went forward and whenever she felt pain, her fist and jaw clenched, she said, "Shit!" and a flash of anger would come over her. On the left side her skin was soft and spongy, her shoulder was back and pain would result in her melting, often followed by tears. The pain was much greater on her left. The overall appearance was of the tough, male, right side protecting the soft, feminine, fragile, left side. This matched her position in the world, where she was a professionally successful woman of great femininity. She turned on one side or the other.[10]

The right/left split can be seen in the way we shape our muscles and tissue, in the way we move and use our body parts, and in the way we nonverbally express and communicate our attitudes and emotions. It is important to keep this separation in mind, for as we crisscross the bodymind and isolate specific regions and limbs, this particular duality will help to pinpoint more specifically the blocks and character traits that animate our bodyminds. In the case of one's hands, for example, which have to do with reaching out and making contact, the left hand is associated with reaching out in a passive, receptive way and the right hand corresponds to reaching out in an active, aggressive fashion.

I am continually asked if there is any relationship between personality style and whether a person is right- or left-handed. As eager as I am to answer this question, I have never been able to come up with any thoroughly convincing evidence that suggests that right- or left-handedness indicates anything other than an individual's muscular and motor preference. While it is true that most people develop their bodies more on the side that they use more actively, the psychological aspects of this split remain unchanged, so that no matter which side they use more comfortably, the right side is still animated by the "masculine" assertive qualities and the left side by the "feminine" receptive forces.

Lately I have heard some interesting information that sheds new light on the relationship between psychological attitudes and right- or left-handedness. The material is part of a study by Dr. Danielle Rapoport[11] on the childbirth techniques of Frederick Leboyer.[12]

Dr. Leboyer is a French obstetrician who has been developing a radically humanistic method of child delivery, focused around creating a birth environment that will be comfortable and pleasant not only for the doctor and mother but, most important, for the child. Dr. Leboyer believes that most hospital births take place amidst insensitivity and violence, harsh lights and sounds, aggressive actions and movements, showing a brutal disregard for the newborn's needs. Leboyer's premise has been that a child born under these conditions, as most of us have been, will immediately armor himself against the insensitivities being perpetrated against him. His further assumption is that a child who begins his life in the presence of such overt insensitivity and violence could possibly adopt an attitude of aggression (or of withdrawal, which in many instances is a form of passive aggression) in response to the harshness of his environment. With respect to the right/left split, this suggests that we very early develop a preference for one side over the other and for the right (assertive) side in most cases, as an expression of an emotional attitude that we developed during our first few moments of life.

Leboyer's technique involves soft lights, gentle handling, delayed umbilicus separation, and mild massage and stroking of the baby by the mother immediately after birth. This process is said to exemplify "birth without violence." Leboyer has been delivering babies in this fashion for more than ten years, and the surprising information that emerges from Rapoport's recent study of these children, besides the fact that they all seem unusually healthy and well adjusted, is that nearly all of them are ambidextrous and seem to display a balanced relationship between the muscles of the right sides of their bodies and those of the left. When I first read this material, I speculated that we might develop preferences for one side over the other because of the attitudes we develop early in life regarding aggression, attitudes that became deeply fixed into our psychosomatic functioning.

Top/Bottom Split

Another major psychosomatic separation in the bodymind is that which is reflected in the top and bottom halves of the body. In many people this split tends to be more dramatic and obvious than is the right/left split.

The bottom half of the bodymind, functionally perceived, is the part of the organism that makes contact with the earth. It is concerned with stabilizing, moving, balancing, supporting, rooting, and establishing a comfortable condition of groundedness. The top half of the bodymind, on the other hand, has to do with seeing, hearing, speaking, thinking, expressing, stroking, hitting, holding, communicating, and breathing.

When perceived psychosocially, the bottom half is oriented toward privacy, support, introspection, homey-ness, emotional stability, dependency, and motion/stasis. The top half is concerned with socializing, outward expression, interpersonal communications and manipulation, self-assertion, aspirations, and action.

One of the easiest ways to tell how a person relates to these aspects of his life is to observe the way his weight is distributed throughout his body. When diagnosing the bodymind in this fashion, it is important to remember that an individual must be viewed with respect to himself and to the way he is proportionately structured, rather than, for example, by having his top half compared with another individual's top half. Each person must be explored in his "wholeness," for it is from that wholeness that the unique personality emerges.

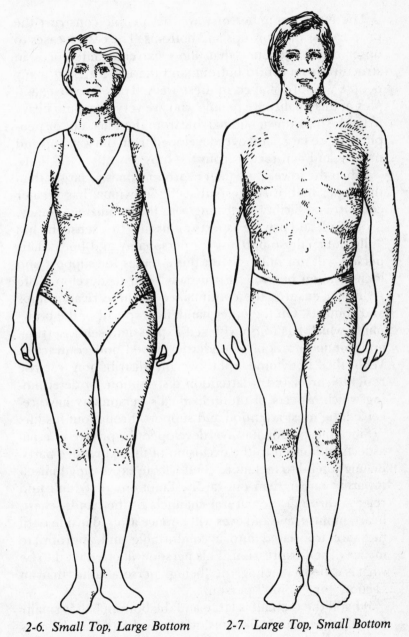

2-6. *Small Top, Large Bottom*   2-7. *Large Top, Small Bottom*

There are a number of ways that people construct the proportions of their tops and bottoms. The easiest cases to observe are the ones that show extreme differences in structure from top to bottom, and there are a great many people who are shaped in these ways. The extreme examples of this duality are people who are very large and heavy from the hips down and narrow from the waist up, or people who are large and overdeveloped from the waist up and narrow and contracted from the hips down.

When the lower body half is proportionately larger than the upper half, it suggests that the individual has greater comfort and facility in dealing with the stabilizing, homey, grounded, and private aspects of his life. In a sense, he has "filled out" these parts of his personality and body. This person will not only rely on these forces for support and identification but will also usually tend to develop a life style that ensures the continuance of these relationships and contacts. On the other hand, the top half of the body-mind, which has to do with self-expression, self-assertion, and communication, is underdeveloped and contracted. With this bodymind split, weight distribution can be roughly correlated to attention distribution, in determining which aspects of the individual's personality have received the most attention and support throughout his life.

Since this person has overdeveloped the private internal aspects of himself to the exclusion of the expressive parts, he might tend to feel more comfortable expressing himself inwardly rather than outwardly. Emotions that can't find release through the natural channels of the hands, chest, heart, mouth, jaw, and eyes will bounce around inside until they are translated into a comfortable and appropriate means of self-expression. This person will often tend to be what is called a "feeling" or "being" person, rather than an "action" or "doing" person.

What if the top half is large and the bottom half is small? We all know people like this, who have large barrel chests and skinny legs with contracted backsides. This person will be overdeveloped in his ability to be expressive, social, assertive, and outgoing, but his thin legs and hips will reflect a lack of strength and fortitude with respect to emotional stability and self-support. As a result, he will have to "stand his ground" with his back, chest, and head, which are his active, assertive aspects, to compensate for the weakness in his legs and emotional roots. This person will probably be more of a mover than a homebody, more prone to action than to stasis. This bodymind type is well illustrated in the following description offered by Alexander Lowen:

> I treated a patient some years ago who suffered severe hypertension. He had been a press agent for several Hollywood stars and movie producers. He was a good eater, a fairly heavy drinker and a smooth talker. He had a round florid face and a full body. When he took his clothes off, I was shocked at the pair of spindly legs and narrow hips that were revealed. The conclusion was inevitable that the seeming security and strength of the upper half of the body was a compensation for the weakness below. His main activities were confined to the upper half of the body and were essentially oral in nature.[13]

These two bodymind extremes are located on opposite ends of a long continuum that includes the whole spectrum of top/bottom possibilities. While very few people fit into these descriptive extremes, most of us do lean in one of the two directions. The degree to which we prefer one style of being over the other is reflected in the amount of top/bottom balance in our bodyminds.

While weight distribution is the most obvious manifestation of this major split, preferences and imbalances can also be detected through other means. For example, the half of the bodymind that is most conscious and developed will usually be more aware and graceful than the other. If a person is talented and coordinated in his upper body and awkward in his legs and hips, he is probably more involved in the aspects of his life that the upper body reflects. Conversely, healthy, active legs accompanied by a stiff or rigid back with clumsy arms suggests an overemphasis on the lower-body aspects of living.

Localized awareness can also be observed in the specific health and vitality of the bodymind halves. In general, it seems that the half of the bodymind that is most graceful and alive will suffer from the fewest dis-eases and injuries, while the half that is rigid and unintegrated, reflecting undeveloped bodymind awareness there, will have suffered from stresses, strains, and injuries.[14] For example, the person with the greater emphasis on the lower bodymind half might suffer from tension headaches, nervous stomach, asthma, or arthritis of the wrists. On the other hand, under-development of the lower half might be reflected in sprained ankles, varicose veins, sexual dysfunction, or flat feet.

It is almost as though we are all made up of two different people, stacked double-decker; the one on the bottom is quiet, shy, reserved, and concerned with being well grounded and emotionally secure; the one on top is outward, assertive, expressive, and concerned with achievement and action. The relationship between these two complementary life forces is reflected in the degree to which these two people relate to each other within ourselves. The same awareness-health/tension—dis-ease relationship also exists with respect to the right/left split. Therefore, you can more accurately pinpoint places of health or dis-ease by further breaking the bodymind down into quadrants, based on the top/bottom, right/left descriptions.

For example, let's say that a person has difficulty making contact with other people because he finds it hard to be assertive. Since he has trouble actualizing his feelings through his arms, we might expect that he would hold the tension in his right arm. If the same person were to have difficulty reaching out to others in a receptive or passive way, the tension would probably localize itself in the left arm. This tension might be manifested as weakness in the joints, tight muscles, or a proneness to injury in this body-mind region.

Or let's say that this person has difficulty "taking a stand." If he is customarily very passive, we might expect the tension to show up somewhere in his right leg. Conversely, if this individual were to have conflicts regarding his ability to take a stand in a receptive fashion, we might expect him to experience tension somewhere in his left leg. These are simple examples of how the right/left and top/bottom splits can be cross-referenced in order to diagnose the bodymind more comprehensively. I will present a more detailed explanation of the apparent relationship between personality and health/dis-ease/growth in the next chapter.

It is important to remember that there is no bodymind structure that is the "right" one. Some people have large tops and small bottoms, others have small tops and large bottoms, others have equally balanced tops and bottoms. Some people injure themselves all the time while others remain healthy and unblemished throughout their lives. Each body is reflective of a unique person with his own unique style of being. Therefore, what is most important about this information, no matter what your particular shape happens to be, is that you realize that your bodymind is made up of many different components and that some of these different preferences and qualities will be reflected in the structure and functions of the top and bottom halves as well as the right and left halves of your bodymind.

In order to appreciate more fully the concept I am presenting here, that we each create our own bodyminds to accommodate the worlds and life styles we have chosen for ourselves, we might compare our life styles to positions we

would play if we were on a football team. Each member of
a football team usually gravitates toward a position on the
team that most appropriately fits his unique size, strength,
skills, and abilities. In addition, each member of the team
will work out and exercise in such a way as to develop and
strengthen the particular muscles and abilities that he will
need in order to play that position most fruitfully and satisfyingly. Similarly, it seems that we all, in the course of our
normal day-to-day living, work out and develop ourselves
with our working, playing, and creating. And in terms of
the entire team of people with whom we play, we each seem
to gravitate toward the position and responsibilities that
most appropriately match our experience, strength, skills,
passions, and abilities. So all the working out and practicing we do, whether it is purely physical or purely emotional,
tend to mold our bodyminds in ways that are simultaneously expressive and definitive of ourselves and our unique
life positions.

Front/Back Split

The third major psychosomatic separation is that of
the front and back sides of the bodymind. Different emotions and psychological attitudes seem to animate these
two sides naturally. The front side appears to reflect the
social self, the conscious self. It is what I knowlingly present
to you; it is what I usually identify as "me." It is the side
of me that I see most often, the side I buy clothing to suit,
and the side of me that I relate to most intimately. It is quite
literally my "front." This side appears to be primarily responsible for those aspects of myself that I am aware of and
that are active ingredients in my day-to-day living: sadness,
happiness, longing, caring, loving, communicating, desir-
ing, are all emotional fields that activate motion and development in the front of my bodymind.

The back side of my bodymind, on the other hand, re-flects the private and unconscious elements of my self. This side often becomes the storehouse for all the aspects of my life that I don't want to deal with or that I don't want other people to see. As a result, I literally place these attitudes and feelings behind me. Quite a bit of unwanted emotion, especially so-called "negative" emotion, gets stored and hidden in the back of my bodymind—along my spine and in the backs of my legs.

It's important to mention briefly that when we experi-ence emotions that we don't want to acknowledge or ex-press, they do not just disappear. We like to think that we can instantaneously remodel everything; so when there is something about our lives that we don't like, we believe that we can have it removed or make it dissolve.

I often feel that many of my patients would like me to be a kind of psycho-roto-rooter man. They'd like to come to me, pay me the necessary money, and have me exorcise the garbage and pain that live within them, blocking the flow of life and happiness. They assume that whatever they are carrying that is "negative" can simply be removed, like sewage from a pipe, or can be covered up with newspaper and made to disappear. But nothing can be simply de-tached and removed from the bodymind. Things can only be moved around or made to change form. So when I work with people, I try to transform their unmentionables into mentionables, bringing what they have put back out of sight into the forefront, into view. Our unwanted garbage can serve as terrific fertilizer.[15]

While it is possible for the back side of the bodymind to be weaker and less congested than the front, it is usually the other way around, as many of our most powerful emotions, such as anger and fear, wind up being stored in the back of the bodymind. As a result, an imbalance is created be-tween the front and back of ourselves, which often leaves the front somewhat too vulnerable and lacking in fortitude while the back becomes a dynamo of overcongested strength and force.

I remember being fascinated by the bodymind of a young man who was in an encounter therapy group that I conducted in Bethlehem, Pennsylvania, in 1972. His body reflected the front/back seperation in a very dramatic way. His front side was soft and tender and sensitive. The muscles in his chest and abdomen were slightly underdeveloped. Seeing him from the front gave the immediate impression that he was a shy, caring, gentle man. When he turned around, however, what you saw was a back that was totally muscular and tight all the way from his neck to his ankles.

When the group began, his actions were consistent with the way his front, or social self, appeared. That is, he was very kind, concerned, and somewhat withdrawn from the major flow of the group. After several days of his very shy behavior one of the other members approached him and accused him of holding back from really opening up to us. The man quietly responded that this was not true, but the pushing and probing continued. After about twenty minutes of trying to get him to come out a bit and reveal himself, something quite unusual happened. This young man shifted abruptly from being quiet and shy to being suddenly wild and ferocious. The Jekyll-to-Hyde transformation was shocking to all of us. It was as though we had all finally gotten around behind him to see what he was holding back and keeping out of our sight with all his politeness and niceties. Not only was he angry with the group, but for nearly forty minutes he screamed and raged about his wife, his boss, his parents, and his children. It was interesting to note that after he had released all of this pent-up energy, his chest relaxed and expanded, and his back and hamstring muscles softened; there was now a closer, healthier balance between his front and back sides. His front and back had shown the same schism in personality that his emotional performance illustrated.

In instances such as this, the front of the bodymind becomes like the living room of a house, with everything arranged just right to present the appropriate social image, while the back is like the attic or basement, jammed with memories, junk, and valuable remnants. In many cases, these hidden and unexpressed feelings and attitudes become frozen into the structure of the body and manifest themselves as tension, stress, and muscular armor, which only serve to further restrict the flow of life throughout the bodymind.

Head/Body Split

The next major psychosomatic separation that I will identify here is the split between the head and the rest of the body. This split is one that we are all probably aware of, and manifests itself on several levels. First, the head and face are our most social aspects. Together they make up the mask that we present to the world. The head and the face are not covered, as the rest of the body usually is, and are used for direct contact and communication more than any other part of the body. The body below the neck, therefore, is more private than above the neck, and, as a rule, most of us are less conscious of it than we are of our heads, because we focus more attention on our faces and intellects than on any other place in the bodymind.

In addition, we Westerners consider the head to be the resting place for the mind, the intellect, and reason. The body, on the other hand, is considered to be our emotional, animal, and less creative aspect. So the obvious splits of body/mind, intellect/feelings, and reason/intuition can all be seen in the way that the head and body relate to each other.

Of all the major bodymind splits, I believe that the one

between the head and the rest of the body is frequently the most pronounced and the most destructive in its relation to the entire human organism. Because of its importance, I will be discussing it in greater detail later in this book, in Chapter 8, on the neck, throat, and jaw.

Torso/Limbs Split

The last major split that I have observed within the bodymind is that between the torso and limbs. This particular split is more difficult to detect than the others but is nevertheless worth discussing briefly. Your torso is the part of your body that can be compared to the "core" of your self. It corresponds to those aspects of your self that are most self-serving, self-reflecting, self-understanding, and self-protecting. In general, it can be said to focus around your "being," as opposed to your limbs, which are more concerned with your "doing." Although the torso is obviously an integrated part of the entire bodymind, I have come to view it as a kind of womb into which we may on occasion retreat. When this happens, it is as though we simply withdraw our aliveness and consciousness from our limbs and periphery and protect ourselves within the confines of our "core."

Our limbs, on the other hand, are those parts of ourselves that we extend from our centers or cores outward into the world in order to perform the functions of moving, acting, making contact, manipulating, and communicating. As a result, our limbs can be thought of as psychosomatic probes that allow us to reach out and expand ourselves past the self-contained limits and restrictions imposed by our torsos. As we take a stand in the world, as we grow outward toward our dreams, and as we reach out and contact other people, we begin to generate our feelings and energy outward into the periphery of our bodyminds through the psychophysical functions of our arms and legs. As I will explain in greater detail later in this book, our legs extend downward from our pelvis to ground us with the earth while our arms extend outward from our chest and shoulders to connect us to people, things, and activities.

The two most obvious examples of the torso/limbs split are that in which the arms and legs are weak and impotent while the torso is full and well developed and that in which the arms and legs are vital and strong, with the torso being frail and underdeveloped.

The first possibility relates to a situation in which a person has filled himself up with his own feelings and passions but has difficulty expressing or mobilizing himself in order to actualize these feelings. In this case, the individual will often feel "all bottled up." I have begun to notice that a great many people who suffer from migraine headaches seem to display this particular torso/limbs relationship. This would make sense, since during a migraine attack the cardiovascular system, by contracting the capillaries in these zones, sends less blood and energy to the periphery of the body. In turn, the contraction of the capillaries increases the pressure and congestion in the core, which then generates the various symptoms and experiences that constitute an attack. In fact, there is some fascinating evidence emerging from the field of clinical biofeedback that suggests that migraine symptoms can be prevented by teaching the sufferer to extend his energy and awareness outward from his core into his limbs before the onset of the attack.[16] By generating a warming feeling in the hands and feet through a kind of self-hypnosis, the person can cause the capillaries at the periphery of his body to remain fully open, and the migraine attack is thereby diverted.

On the other hand, the individual with a thin torso and overdeveloped arms and legs might tend to be more of a "do-er" than a "be-er." The body of the comic strip character "Popeye" suggests an extreme version of this type of body structure. Whereas the last person that I described would have difficulty "unbottling" himself and allowing his deeply developed core to expand outward into the expressive channels of his limbs, this second person would tend to have difficulty making contact at all with his core, for he is too busy acting out the functions that correspond to his legs and arms. This person will tend to spend more time with other people and activities than he will with himself. In fact, for him, holding still and remaining quiet within himself might be a difficult and uncomfortable activity.[17]

Before I proceed to discuss the psychosomatic nature of the feet, I'd like to ask you to put this book down and once again observe yourself in a full-length mirror. As you look at yourself this time, pay attention to the various bodymind splits that I have just described. See if you can be more aware of any imbalances that exist in your bodymind and allow yourself to relate these imbalances to the corresponding preferences and habits that highlight your character and life style. As you view yourself in this fashion, try to see the parts of your bodymind that are undeveloped not as points of weakness but rather as untapped regions of yourself, to be further explored and developed.

FEET AND LEGS

"RELAX YOUR SHOULDERS, KEN!" "Unlock your knees and allow your legs to move fluidly." "Try to see if you can let yourself move from your belly rather than your chest." "Feel your movements, stop thinking them!" "Relax your muscles so that your body yields to the energy and flow of your movement . . . yield!" "Let your legs support and carry you, not your head, that's what legs are for."

And so went my first T'ai Chi lesson. The above suggestions are only a few of the many pointers on how to use my bodymind more economically and appropriately that Judith Weaver gave me during my lessons. T'ai Chi is an Oriental form of movement/meditation that combines mental concentration, coordination of breathing, and a graceful series of deliberate body movements. It evolved in ancient China as an art of graceful self-defense and took its philosophical base from Taoism, a philosophy that encourages yielding and "going with the flow" rather than aggression and offensive action.

The motions that are employed in T'ai Chi are very un-

like our usual movements in that they are initiated from a
point a few inches below the navel, in the center of the
body. This point is the actual physical center of the body
and is called the "tan tien." Most of us, when we walk and
move, lead with our chest, shoulders, or head. In order to
move from the "tan tien," the T'ai Chi student must learn
to focus a great deal of attention and consciousness on the
lower half of his body in order to compensate for his normally exaggerated attention on the upper half. By securing
himself on the powerful foundation of his legs, he becomes
able to move, yield, and hold ground in a gracefully dynamic way.

In studying T'ai Chi, one must learn to become subtly
aware not only of one's bodymind but also of the way it
moves through the enveloping space. Intense concentration and focus are required in order to perform the T'ai Chi
movements. It is a kind of moving meditation.

In t'ai chi practice, you move very slowly. By moving very
slowly you have time to be aware of all the subtle details of
your movement and your relationship to your surround-
ings. It's so slow that you really have no way of saying this
is slower than that or faster than that. You reach a level of
speed that is like slow motion in which everything is just
happening. You slow it to the point that you are fully involved in the process of each moment as it happens.[1]

I have found that T'ai Chi is a lot like yoga in that it is
a bodymind process that involves a great deal of practice
and self-discipline to master: the T'ai Chi student may
spend years practicing several simple movements before he
reaches a state of awareness of the subtleties of his own
bodymind. Also, like yoga, T'ai Chi allows its practitioners
a means for self-exploration, self-development, and increased awareness. T'ai Chi differs from yoga in that all
movements are performed in a standing position. As a result, there is an incredible amount of emphasis placed on

the legs and the way the bodymind uses the legs to support it against gravity's continual pull. Also, I have found that T'ai Chi, which by heritage belongs to the Oriental martial arts, is considerably more concerned with one's relationship to what is outside of oneself, such as potential attackers, gravity, and air, than is yoga, which focuses almost entirely on one's inner worlds of self-attention, self-reflection, and self-awareness.[2]

When I began studying with Ms. Weaver, she was six months pregnant, so it was easy to follow the motions of her "tan tien" as it protruded about five inches from her body. It was a beautiful sight to watch this pregnant woman move so gently yet so powerfully through the deliberate movements of the T'ai Chi form. Her body seemed so centered, so grounded, and so graceful that I was embarrassed by my own awkwardness in comparison. Yet through my experience with T'ai Chi and with Judith Weaver, I was able to discover several fascinating things about myself that have been a part of me ever since.

My most wonderful discovery through T'ai Chi was that I had legs, and that they not only connected to my pelvis but also continued straight down to the earth. This might sound silly, but in fact I was hardly aware of my legs and how to use them appropriately before my first T'ai Chi lesson. It's almost frightening that I could have gone through twenty years of walking, running, standing, and living without learning how to use my legs to support and motivate myself. I discovered that I had come to use my back for standing (I had overdeveloped my back muscles to compensate for weak leg muscles), my shoulders for walking (I led with my chest and shoulders rather than my legs and belly), and my jaw and eyes for support (to make up for the weakness I experienced in my feet and legs). Through T'ai Chi I began to explore other, more relaxed ways of moving, standing, and being.

As we began the first of the 108 traditional T'ai Chi

movements, Judith continually reminded me to move from my "tan tien," which meant that I would have to relax and lower my center of consciousness to coincide with my center of gravity. This bodymind lowering and centering shifted a great deal of stress and support from my back to my legs and feet. After several frustrating weeks of not being able to make conscious use of my legs, Judith gave me an image that has served as a powerful way for me to alter and improve the entire image I had of my bodymind. She told me to imagine that my legs were roots, and that they not only supported my body but also continued straight down through the surface of the earth as far as I could imagine. She asked me to think of my legs as my history, explaining to me that they possessed the historical foundation upon which my entire being rested. She suggested that if I would allow myself to use my legs in this fashion, I could draw energy up from them and from the earth and that this would help me relax all of the compensatory control I was exercising with the upper portion of my bodymind. It worked. As soon as I visualized my legs in this image, my center of consciousness dropped down from my shoulders to my belly, and I immediately felt more grounded and stable than I had ever felt before.

This powerful image, and the feelings that I experienced when I was able to capture its meaning, are the closest I can come to presenting my own conception of "grounding." This word has become quite popular lately and has taken on a variety of meanings.[3] For me it simply refers to the recognition that the earth is the body from which I have evolved and from which I draw support and stability. My primary contact with the earth comes through my feet and legs, which are my physical contacts with the earth and my psychological foundation. As my body relates to the earth and its gravitational pull, so do I relate to my own sense of psychological stability, as manifested in my ability to be secure and relaxed when I am still, or centered and flexible when I am in motion.

In the rest of this chapter I will be sharing some of my explorations and observations regarding the feet, ankles, knees, and legs. While these parts all have relatively similar psychosomatic functions, there are qualities peculiar to each of them. The discussion is based on my personal and clinical studies and on a variety of related psycho-therapeutic fields and self-exploration disciplines.

THE FEET

Now, look at your feet. That's right, stop reading this page and take a moment to look closely at your feet. Get a mirror, if you need one, and take a good look at your feet. Who are they? What are they shaped like? What do they feel like? Do they provide the appropriate structure upon which you can build the rest of your bodymind?

Are your feet healthy looking? Are your toes curled under? Are your feet colder than the rest of your body? Do they bring you a great deal of pleasure or do they only give

3-1. Healthy Foot, Showing Three Points of Contact with the Ground

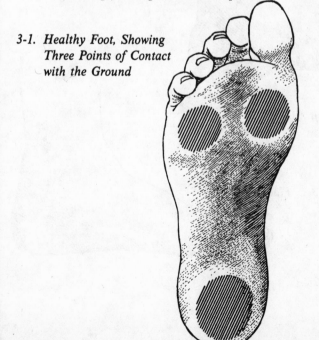

you pain? Do you take good care of your feet? What do they like?

Healthy, unblocked, untwisted feet are platforms with three distinct points of contact and with a sufficient metatarsal arch. If you have flat feet, it means that you have only one interface between each foot and the ground. If you have an exaggerated arch, it means that your feet make contact with the earth at two points.

Feet and the way a person uses them for support and balance are excellent indicators of how stable and grounded the person is, for, as I noted, the way a person is grounded physically is frequently identical to the way he is grounded emotionally. For this reason, there is a lot to

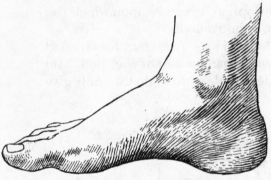

3-2. Healthy, Well-Grounded Foot

3-3. Flat Foot

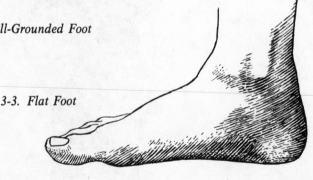

be learned by observing the feet. According to William Schutz, "The feet are of vital importance psychologically because they are the contact with reality, the ground and gravity. Physically, an imbalance at the feet throws off the balance of the total structure."[4] As a result of their structure and function, the feet indicate the chronic stance and attitude that a person needs to assume in order to meet comfortably the challenges of his life. For example, when we speak of a person as being "earthy," we usually mean that he has a good sense of reality, whereas when we say someone is "up in the air" or "flighty," we are indicating that he is out of contact with reality.[5]

The easiest and most obvious way to discuss foot structure and its relationship to personality is through examples, but as I describe these types of feet, it's helpful to remember that we each develop as a total unit, and the feet we create are intimately tied in to the rest of ourselves. It is necessary to present many of the parts before the "wholes" become more obvious to you, however, and as we get more and more involved in seeing the body as the direct reflection of character, the interrelationships between the various bodymind parts and regions will become clearer.

Flat Feet

I had had flat feet for most of my life, so I know well what they are about. Flat feet indicate an ungrounded, "hockey puck" way of relating to the world, both physically as well as psychologically. The hockey-puck-footed person will skid and slide along the surface of the planet, never quite putting down roots, never quite standing still. These feet allow a great deal of ease in motion, but they do not allow the fluidity and stability that would make that ease effective. The disadvantage of this psychosomatic combination is that such a person might have a difficult time staying still in relation to other people and responsibilities, and might be motivated by a nervous need to be in motion rather than by a reason for moving. He might also tend to have an overdeveloped back, neck, and head to accommodate psychosomatically to the lack of stability and support in this lower segment. For this fish, stillness is not the natural water in which he can swim comfortably.

Clutching Feet

There is a simple experiment that you can try by which you can see at once what kind of feet you have. First, find a friend to help you with this experiment. Stand up and assume a position that feels natural and comfortable. Then,

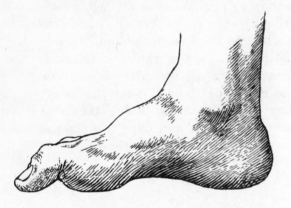

3-4. *Clutching Foot*

3-5. *Heel-Digging Foot*

have your friend gently place his hand on your chest and begin to push. He should push hard enough so that you have to tighten your body in response to his confrontation but not so hard that you might fall over. Next, have him walk around behind you and push again, this time on your back between your shoulder blades. You might also have him try to knock you off your feet by pushing on either side of you. His pushing should be slow and gentle so that, as the pressure of the push builds, you will have to slowly tighten muscles and rear-range your posture to meet the force of his confrontation. As you are responding to the physical pressure, be aware of what parts of your body actively resist being pushed over and how they do this. You might be surprised to find that the attitude that you assume with your entire body, and in particular with your feet, might actually demonstrate the type of psychological posture that you assume when other aspects of your life (such as emotions and beliefs) are similarly confronted.

For example, flat-footed people will usually lose their ground pretty quickly and will be easily pushed off their spot, no matter how heavy or formidable they appear. Clutchers, on the other hand, usually respond to the confrontation by "clutching" with their entire body and most exaggeratedly with their feet. The toes will curl under and the arch will clench in an attempt to grasp the earth and the forces of stability and self-support. Often, clutchers' feet have grown over the years to assume this clenched attitude chronically. When this happens, the muscles of the feet tend to become rigid and chronically tense. Sometimes, the tension in the feet is related to an unresolved emotional crisis that involved the possibility of movement or running away. If the impulse to flee is not acted upon, the muscles of the feet may register the conflict by spastically clenching the earth. This unnatural clutching stance tends to further rigidify and distort the muscles of the feet, thereby locking the conflict into the tissue itself. This possibility was ob-

served by William Schutz while Rolfing a middle-aged man
with rigid feet:

> Another man found great pain in his feet as I worked on
> them [second Rolfing session] and had to keep them mov-
> ing. I asked him to keep them moving until he found out
> what they wanted to do. "Run away," he said, "I want to run
> away." He immediately thought of both his immediate situ-
> ation, in which he was unhappy with his marriage, and his
> early childhood situation, when his father pressured him to
> become a doctor. The feet had evidently prepared them-
> selves for running away many times but had never been able
> to complete the act. The result was great tension in the
> muscles and fasciae of the feet.[6]

When people are forced to hold their ground by squeezing their feet and legs, the rest of the bodymind follows suit
and develops a full bodymind posture that fits in with the
"clutching" style of self-support. These people frequently
have overdeveloped thighs and a correspondingly overemphasized need for self-control to compensate for the lack
of fluid stability and relaxed contact with the earth. Clutchers are frequently tight in the muscles that live in the back
of the body, especially in the back of the legs and knees or
the lower back, all related to an overdeveloped need to
hold on and to keep things under control.

Weight on Heels

This sort of psychosomatic posture seems to express
an exaggerated feeling of determination, which is often
accompanied by a false sense of stability. You might stand
up again and ask your friend to try to push you over once
more. If you respond by "digging in your heels," you probably fit into this general bodymind category. According to
Alexander Lowen: "When the weight of the body is directly
over the heels, the standing position can be upset easily by

a slight push backwards. Here again the common expression describes the situation well. We say of such a person that he is a 'pushover.' "[7]

Because this person is so easily pushed over and manipulated, he may respond, in order to remain stable and grounded, by developing a chronic attitude of determination and control, though this may still be accompanied by deep feelings of fear and instability. For example, when I dig in my heels, I notice that I also unconsciously clench my jaw and tighten my belly, which seems to shorten my breathing. When I hold this position for a little while, I begin to feel anxious and somewhat afraid. As a result of this constant vigilance, the person who digs in his heels will have a hard time relaxing and feeling comfortable in spontaneous situations. The overdeveloped need to dig in and hold on might also be reflected in a constricted chest, a nervous stomach, and especially in a rigid pelvis and lower back.

Tiptoers

We all know people who are tiptoers. When they walk, they seem to be walking mostly on their toes and hardly put any weight at all on their heels. People who walk and stand in this fashion always seem to me to be like fairy princesses or princes. It almost seems that if these people had just a bit more imaginative thrust they would lift themselves off the earth and float away. Surely these people will have a hard time making contact, physically or psychologically, with the forces of the earth. Instead they are often floaters and dreamers, and frequently are highly imaginative and possess artistic abilities.

Lead Feet

People with lead feet seem to have created lives and psychosystems for themselves that keep them weighted down. These people are almost opposite to the tiptoers; floating away presents entirely too much uncertainty and instability for them to handle. For the lead-footed person, there is a strong need to be grounded, to be stable, to know one's position in life. Accompanying this emphasis on stasis is a difficulty in dealing with motion and change. These people are usually more reliable and set than they are creative and active.

Let me just mention that I think it is a great art to be able to plant your weight and energy beneath you in order to be rooted and self-supported. There are many wonderful stories of T'ai Chi and Aikido masters who can ground their energies in such a way that they cannot be moved or lifted off the spot. Similarly, there is a great advantage in being able to hold your intellectual or emotional position when the situation demands.

The dis-ease develops, however, when this holding is generated by chronic fear or anxiety; when you have so forcefully overemphasized your need to be secure and stable that the rest of your bodymind takes on a forced, resistant, or rigid attitude in relation to the flow of life. In this case, lead feet will weigh you down and may encourage stagnation and self-decay.

Most people would argue that their feet are shaped as they are because of hereditary factors or because of the physical activities with which they have been engaged. While these components of bodymind structuring no doubt affect the nature and functioning of the feet, I have been discovering that the psychoemotional components of one's life also seem to be formative in the continual re-creation of this part of the bodymind.

For example, earlier in this section I mentioned that I used to have flat feet. I had always believed that my flat feet were hereditary, because my father also had, and still has, flat feet. As I became more aware of my own bodymind, however, I began to realize that my flat feet had developed as a result of the way that I had come to deal with the continuous challenges of my life, and that the only way that I could change the arches in my feet would be to also change the way that I psychologically ground myself . . . the way I am.

So, for the past three years I have been trying to ground myself in a different way, by becoming more responsible in my interpersonal interactions and by being less scattered in my interests and activities. At first, it was totally against my nature to be this way, and I felt the pressure of a lifetime of emotional inertia pushing me to remain hockey-puckish. I have since come to appreciate more fully the need for balance and stability in my life and have of late been finding it quite easy to slow down and support myself a bit more with my roots and foundation. For me, these changes have been very down-to-earth and mundane; they have involved things like moving into a new and more comfortable house, staying with the same project for over three years, and trying to be more focused in my relationships with family and friends. As a result of these basic life changes, I am not surprised to discover that my arches have increased considerably and that my feet are no longer flat.

Apparently, my way of being in the world had always "fitted" the shape and functional abilities of my feet, which were flat and ungrounded. By changing my life style, I altered my way of being in the world, thereby releasing many of the conflicts and tensions that I had habitually experienced. As I became more grounded, my feet began to change in order to reflect more appropriately the new way I made contact with the earth: they became more grounded too. In trying to improve my ability to ground myself, I might have chosen to restructure my feet in two different ways: through exercises and massage with the hope that new feet would allow a new way of being, or by a change in my life style in the expectation that my feet would gently reshape themselves to accommodate my new psychoemotional patterns. In this instance, I took the second route and met with a pleasant success.

I have also come to see that my father and I both had flat feet not because of our genes but because we shared the same ways of dealing with life. So rather than blame my parents' genes for my structure, I have begun to assume responsibility for the way I am, and this has allowed me the power to change and restructure myself. As long as I placed the responsibility for my condition on something or someone other than myself, there was little possibility for change. As soon as I owned myself, I allowed myself the power of conscious change and creative self-development.

Before I move on to discuss the ankles and knees, I would like to briefly discuss a form of bodymind diagnosis and healing that relates specifically to the health and well-being of the feet. "Foot reflexology," or "zone therapy," as it is sometimes called, has become an increasingly popular practice in the last few years. "Foot reflexology" recognizes the feet to be important indicators of the health/dis-ease of the entire bodymind system.[8] The theory behind reflexology is that for every organ or major muscle area in the trunk and head, there is a tiny area that corresponds to it on the feet. If the body part is healthy and well functioning, the corresponding area of the feet is also healthy and well functioning. If the specific body part is toxic or unhealthy, the corresponding point on the feet will be similarly toxic —and very sensitive to touch.

You might take a moment to examine your feet by slowly exploring them with your fingers, pressing firmly as you go, and paying attention to whether or not you feel pain or soreness at various points. Then, refer to the reflexology charts on pages 62–63 to see exactly which body parts relate to the areas of soreness that you discovered. Within the reflexology system, it is believed that the way to restore vitality and health to any particular body organ or region is to gently and regularly massage the corresponding areas of the feet. When the body part is restored to health, the foot tenderness will disappear; conversely, when you have massaged all of the soreness out of your feet, the related body part should be well. A healthy body is therefore reflected in healthy, vital feet.

There are several complementary theories to explain why this is true. One theory is focused on the flow of lymph in the body. Lymph is the fluid that purifies the blood, enhancing the general health of the body. The lymph fluid circulates throughout the body picking up debris and dead cells and then returns this garbage to the heart. Often, this matter gets trapped and blocked at the areas called "lymph nodes." Stimulation of these nodes encourages further breakdown of the refuse and adds to the vitalization of the body. There are numerous lymph nodes in the feet, and for this reason it is believed that reflexology works primarily through the lymphatic system.

Another theory has to do with what the Chinese call "chi" energy. This subtle energy flows throughout the body along paths that are called "meridians," and the healthy flow and balance of this energy are responsible for the health conditions of the organism. All the meridians have terminal points in the feet, roughly corresponding to the lymph nodes that are there. By massaging these points, a healthy flow of energy is encouraged, thus restoring balance and vitality to the body.[9]

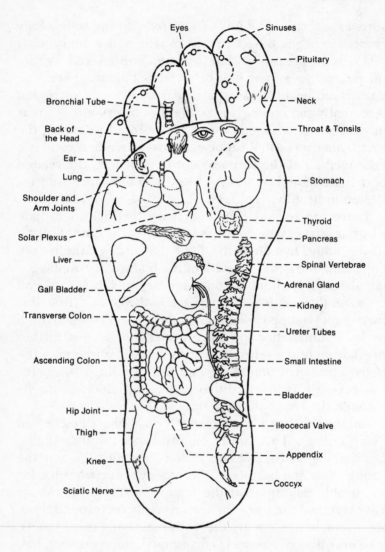

3-6. Foot Reflexology Chart: Right Foot

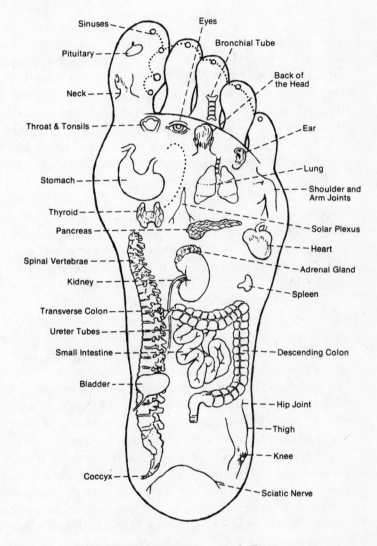

3-7. Foot Reflexology Chart: Left Foot

THE ANKLES AND KNEES

The ankles and knees are joints (the ankle is a ball-and-socket, the knee is a hinge), and all joints are psychosomatic crossroads. As crossroads, they have to mediate between the forces, physical as well as psychological, that flow through them. I believe that it is the quality of our joints that allows us to be either graceful and well integrated or spastic and disjointed. For this reason, the psychosomatic condition of the joints reveals a great deal about the way an individual is dealing with the flow and motion of his life. In addition, when these crossroads have traffic jams and roadblocks too often, they can become chronically tense and blocked, thereby interrupting the flow of life that runs through them. When this happens, the joints not only lose their flexibility and grace but can also become extremely susceptible to injury and dis-ease. The health and stability of the ankles and knees is especially critical, for they are in positions that demand that they continually support the entire bodymind against the continuous pull of the earth.

Psychosomatically, the ankles and knees are related to many of the same character traits and qualities that were attributed to the feet, such as stability, grounding, contact with the earth, ease of movement and change, self-support, and a sense of ease and presence. In addition, I have discovered during my years as an athletic instructor and a yoga teacher that injuries to the ankles and knees are frequently related to psychological conflicts around feelings relating to how a person is dealing with progress or resistance to progress. I have been fascinated to observe that in many cases of ankle or knee injury, the individuals were involved in a considerable degree of personal tension concerning this aspect of their lives.

It might be said, therefore, that the knees and ankles reflect the sense of ease with which we progress through our lives and move through the world. When these aspects of our lives are flowing and open, our ankles and knees are flexible and vital; when we are stuck, or tentative or conflicted, our ankles and knees will have a tendency to rigidify and thereby become more susceptible to injury.

HEALTH, DIS-EASE, AND PERSONAL GROWTH

It would probably be helpful at this point if I shared some of my beliefs and feelings in regard to injuries and dis-eases of the bodymind. It is appropriate that I use the knees as examples for this discussion, for I have recently had a great deal of trouble with my left knee, troubles that culminated in a torn cartilage and its subsequent surgical removal.

Throughout my life I have always been active athletically. I have also been reckless in the way I have treated my bodymind while engaged in these activities. As a result, I have suffered my share of sprains, twists, pulls, and breaks. As I look back, I notice that most of these injuries occurred at joints or right near them. In particular, most of these so-called accidents affected either my ankles or knees. I had always believed that these injuries occurred because so-and-so pushed me, or because I fell the wrong way, or because the floor on which I was running was slippery. Lately, as I have become more aware of my own psychosomatic nature and have begun to take greater responsibility for more of my actions, I have noticed that all my injuries have occurred at times and at bodymind locations of extreme psychosomatic stress; the locations therefore offered a lowered threshold of vitality to the activity and aggressive movement I was involved in.[10]

The most recent of the injuries to my knee occurred in March 1974, after many injury-less years of preventive health maintenance. After the initial injury and prior to the corrective operation, I experienced nine months of intermittent pain and annoyance which kept me continually

aware of and sensitive to the needs of my knee. Anyone who
has ever sprained an ankle or twisted a wrist knows what it
is like to have such an important part of your body not
working up to its previous capacities. I had a chance to
learn a great deal about myself during those months, however, and I found that the added attention to my knee
allowed me to begin to see exactly what was happening in
there and why I damaged it in the first place. It is too bad
that I didn't have this information clear in my bodymind
before the time of the injury.

It is primarily through my yoga studies that I have
evolved a simple and worthwhile way of looking at my
injury—and at all injuries, for that matter—a way that has
allowed me to gain a great deal of insight into my own
health/dis-ease processes. This yogic explanation of health
and dis-ease, which I shall briefly explain, offers a considerably different perspective on health and stress than the one
that we have learned from our contemporary medical system, and I believe that in some ways it is a more appropriate
means of understanding the way that the bodymind develops, functions, and malfunctions.

The word *yoga* derives from the word *yuj* and is roughly
translated to mean "yoke," or "union." The implication is
that through the yogic exploration of himself, an individual
can achieve a state of union with himself and with the universe of which he is a part.

There are four primary yogic paths: karma yoga, which
is the way of action; bhakti yoga, which is the yoga of devotion and selfless love; jnana (or gnani) yoga, which is
the path of self-reflection and wisdom, the philosophical
yoga; and raja yoga, which is considered the "kingly
yoga."[11] Raja yoga contains elements of the other three
yoga paths but is primarily characterized by techniques of
physical exercise, meditation, and pranayama (breathing
exercises). Raja is the form of yoga that most of us are
familiar with. Since this branch of yoga is concerned with

physical, mental, and emotional development, it includes a variety of well-known bodymind disciplines such as hatha yoga, prana yoga, tantric yoga, Kundalini yoga, and siddha yoga.

I have been practicing hatha yoga and jnana yoga since 1968. Although hatha and jnana yoga deal with different aspects of self-knowledge, I have discovered that when they are explored and translated through the bodymind, they begin to emerge as nearly identical expressions of the same basic knowledge. I will try to share a bit of this perspective with you.

The yoga perspective recognizes that each of us is made up of a great many forces, feelings, limits, possibilities, and passions. These aspects exist within my body and my mind and collectively define the boundaries that I usually identify as "me." Physically, these limits are experienced as muscle tension, restricted movement, and pain. Psychologically, limits are experienced as dogma, ignorance, and fear. Most limits have the potential to continually change and restructure themselves.

Now, if I sit on the floor and try to reach over to touch my toes, I might notice that I can only stretch to about five inches away from my toes before I experience tension and slight pain. At this point, the muscles in my lower back and the muscles in the back of my legs are just too tight to allow me any further stretch. At this point I am experiencing one of my boundaries.

This point, this "edge," is a highly important place, for within the yogic philosophy, this edge is considered to be my creative teacher from whom I can learn about myself. If I approach this teacher/edge with love, sensitivity, and awareness, I will discover that my teacher/edge will move and allow me a greater range of motion. If I shy away from approaching my teacher/edge, I will learn nothing new, and in time my own dogma/tightness will contract upon itself and I will grow even tighter. If I try to blast past my edge, I might fool myself into thinking that I have learned and expanded, but in fact what usually happens is that I am only impressing myself with a temporary surge of ambition and that this feeling will probably contract upon itself with fear and subsequent tightening, forcing me into greater confusion or potentially dangerous misunderstandings. Physically, when I approach my edge gently and consciously, my body responds by focusing energy and attention on this spot, encouraging the blood and energy to bathe the related muscles and organs with vitality and life, thus allowing me the experience of true growth and self-nourishment. But if I do not try to reach my edge, my body, having no point of focus, will find it difficult to isolate the place and nourish it, and little growth and improvement will follow.

To state the extremes: If I never explore my limits, my bodymind will gradually tighten and become unconscious. If I regularly explore my limits in a caring and adventuresome fashion, I will expand and grow in a vital fashion. But if I try to push myself past where I am honestly able to go, I will not longer be practicing "yoga" but instead will be practicing "greed," and I will probably be met by pain and disease. Stated simply, it is the difference between *ignoring* your self, *making love* to yourself, and *raping* yourself.

The other fascinating aspect is that the teacher/edge, in addition to defining the limits of expansion and contraction, also distinguishes the fine line that exists between self-destruction and self-improvement. Thus, the artist continually strives to reach deeper past his own abilities and limits in order to experience a new idea, a creative insight, or an illuminating vision. But if he pushes himself past his own limits too fast or too hard, he might experience tension, pain, and suffering. And so will the athlete or yogi who does the same. When psychological or physical growth are pushed too hard, the movement toward expansion and growth is often forced to take a side turn into the domain of pain, stress, and discomfort.

Now, what does all of this have to do with health, dis-ease, and personal growth? Well, the implication of this yogic perspective is that health, dis-ease, and personal growth are all aspects of the way in which you deal with yourself. When you are being loving to yourself and are without chronically painful conflicts, your bodymind will manifest a state of health. Similarly, when you are being unconscious and unloving toward yourself, you run the risk of moving your bodymind into a state of dis-ease and stress, which could undermine your health and hamper your growth. This perspective also suggests that the most effective and efficient way to develop yourself is to be as mindful and as aware as possible, all the while being respectful of self-limits and appreciative of continually regenerating expansiveness.

This perspective reflects the yogic nonviolent, noncompetitive, holistic approach to growth, education, and health, in contrast to our Western philosophy and health practices, which are often competitive, aggressive, and self-insensitive.[12]

When the bodymind deals with itself in an insensitive fashion, it often causes injury, strain, and malfunction, and the specific location of the dis-ease is usually an excellent indication of the exact sort of uncaring aggressiveness that it has been enacting upon itself.

A perfect example of how bodymind stress leads to injury and psychosomatic dis-ease can be observed in the factors that contributed to my tearing the cartilage in my left knee. Several years ago, I was living peacefully in Big Sur, California, in a small cabin surrounded by a redwood forest. I had been living there for nearly two years, and my life had become comfortable and set. One morning, my landlord knocked on my door and woke me up to tell me that he had decided to let several close friends of his live in my house and that I would have to move out within a few days. I was instantly and totally unhappy about this unexpected change in my life.

I had many conflicting questions. Should I stay in Big Sur or should I leave? If I left, where should I go and why should I go there? At that time, my professional life was reaching a critical stage that had me confronting my own escalating popularity within the human-potential movement. Needless to say, my own ego and ambitions were embarrassingly in motion. I was scheduled to begin a six-week lecture/workshop tour on the East Coast in four weeks, so I moved all my things out of my house and placed them and me on a friend's doorstep until it was time to fly to New York. I was so rattled by having to leave and pack up all of my lovely house into boxes that my yoga practice suffered badly and my body grew stiff.

While on the East Coast, my mind tossed and turned with impending life decisions, keeping me partially ungrounded wherever I was. My thoughts were filled with insecurity, and my bodymind was forced to experience and store all this unresolved stress.

So, my self-stability, ego, and aggressiveness were all in a state of conflict, and the conflict manifested in my knees, especially in my left knee, which was trying to tell me to slow down. If I had been paying attention to myself, I might have responded to these signals and might have been able to balance all the confusions alive in my bodymind, but as is usually the case in situations of turmoil, I was even less mindful than usual. So, one day when I was doing my daily exercises, I decided to boost my ego by trying to perform an extremely difficult yoga posture that I had only achieved several times before in my life.

This posture demanded that I push a great many of my muscle regions to their limits at the same time, causing a kind of consciousness-juggling act within my own psychophysical system. The area of least awareness and greatest stress, my left knee, simply would not bear the strain of so much psychosomatic stress. My knee gave way, and I tore the medical meniscus cartilage on the inside of my left knee.

If I suspend all value judgments as to the goodness or badness of injuries, I can clearly see that this injury provided a clear statement of the condition of my bodymind at that point in my life. With a kind of physical scream, it reminded me of who and what I was at that particular instant. The crazy thing about injuries is that they often force us finally to pay attention to ourselves.

As soon as I felt the tear and the pain, I painfully recognized that I had been unconscious of myself for weeks. The pain in my knee brought me back to an awareness of my self-responsibility. Although upset about the injury, I was strangely pleased about the closeness I once again felt with myself. I am not suggesting that everyone should go out and tear his body apart in order to get to know it. I am proposing, however, that the bodymind demands and deserves attention and self-appreciation and that when it is neglected or distressed, it becomes more susceptible to stress and injury. In my own case, the point of dis-ease was exactly at the crossroads that most explicitly illustrated my state of stress at that time in my life. During such times of conflict, concentrated attention is needed in order to maintain bodymind harmony, yet many of us usually pay *less* loving attention to ourselves during these periods of turmoil and stress.

This example from my own life is one in which an acute injury grew out of unrecognized and uncared-for chronic stress. The blockage was the manifestation of all the unresolved factors in my life and all the feelings I had within me in regard to these factors. So, this injury was not something that happened to me over which I had no control. Nor was it an accident. Rather, it was an honest and accurate

statement of what I was doing with and to myself that was
simply being reflected back to me through the language of
my bodymind. Since this knee injury, and because of my
growing realization that the functioning of my bodymind is
related to my own inner states of harmony and health, I
have become much more in tune with the needs of my
bodymind and thereby much more able to mindfully and
lovingly heal and harmonize the variety of forces and passions that exist within it . . . within me.

While your bodymind is a remarkably efficient and dura-
ble self-healing machine, it has its limits.[13] If the psychosomatic edges are uncared for or exploited, your bodymind
will experience tension, stress, pain, illness, injury, and
eventual self-destruction. I have come to believe that bodymind malfunctions usually occur at times of stress and at
psychosomatic locations that are engaged in stressful interactions to the point that the healthy threshold for dis-
ease has been lowered, thereby allowing weakness or ill
health to occur. For instance, when a part of the bodymind
is held tight, separated from the flow of energy and nourishment that regularly courses through the body, that region will tend to malfunction and die first. If you placed one
hundred flowers in a room and denied ten of them light and
water, the ten would die first. So it is in the human bodymind; regions of unresolved conflict can become barren
psychosomatic deserts existing within an otherwise vital
ecosystem. The areas that are choked of life and energy will
become less vital, more fragile, more dis-eased, and therefore more prone to injury and sickness.

Points of psychosomatic stress can turn up anywhere in
the bodymind. In the belly, they might show up as a spastic
colon or as a cyst on an ovary; in the chest, they might
manifest as a chest cold, as asthma, or as a bronchial attack;
in the pelvis, tension and blockage might appear as sexual
frigidity or as a sciatic condition; in the neck, the conflict
may be felt as tension and limited movement. Or conflicts

may turn up at the joints, because, as I have mentioned, the joints are crossroads and are therefore extremely suscepti-ble to blockage and conflict.

Thus, sickness and injury can be appreciated as warning signals, nonverbal messages that your body transmits when you are not taking appropriate care of yourself. If you can learn to translate these somatic messages into psychoemo-tional information, you can be more aware of your needs, passions, and conflicts. In this sense, the bodymind is its own problem solver, with the wrong answers showing up as tension and the right answers showing up as vitality.

For example, since I have become aware that my knees get tight and rigid when I am confused and ungrounded, I have begun to exercise my knees with T'ai Chi and yoga each day in order to insure myself against the occurrence of these feelings. I have found that when I keep the en-ergy flowing freely through my legs, it is much more diffi-cult for me to feel shaky and uncertain. Similarly, when I discover that my legs are unusually tight and that my knees are more rigid than usual, I take this information as a sign that I am moving too unconsciously through my life. If my left knee is the tense one, as it was before my injury, I try to slow down my pace and become more pas-sive. If my right knee is problematic, I try to become more assertive and active with my intellectual, emotional, and physical activities. In this way, I have come to know how to use myself more effectively in my daily activities and decision-making processes.

When blockages to growth and health manifest in your physical body, you feel them as pain and dis-ease; similar conflict in the psychoemotional realm will appear as unhap-piness, anxiety, depression, and neurotic behavior. The trick is to become so aware of and so intimate with yourself that you can catch these signals and messages before they become destructive and irreversible. The mindful individ-ual learns to listen to every cell in his bodymind and to be

responsive to its needs and lessons. This is one of the aims
of yoga.

By learning how to avoid dis-ease and emotional problems, we can also begin to aim ourselves toward conditions
of super-health and continued emotional happiness. It is
almost as though we have to learn how to be healthy and
happy and that these skills must be regularly practiced to
assure their continuance.

THE LEGS

While very few people ever actually injure their knees, all
of us frequently hold tension and stress in our legs that to
some degree impairs our movements and limits our bodymind awareness. For example, stand up and experience
your legs. Imagine that you are in an extremely desirable
situation and that you are really happy about being there.
Feel grounded and secure. As you feel these possibilities,
be aware of your legs and get a sense for the way they feel
to you.

Now imagine that you are in a totally undesirable situation and that what you would like most of all to do would
be to leave, to run away. With these feelings present in your
mind, be aware of your legs. Do they feel any different?

Chances are you felt yourself tighten up either at the
knees and ankles or in your thighs and hamstring muscles.
Either way, it should be obvious to you that when you felt
as though you wanted to be somewhere else, either physically or psychologically, some part or parts of your legs
responded by registering the conflict. The conflict manifests itself in the form of tension, and the tension will continue to live in the related parts of your legs chronically,
unless it is released.

Or imagine that you are in some position or situation that
you especially enjoy and are afraid that someone might
come along and force you to leave or else somehow ruin it

for you. Try to feel what response you might have to being taken away from something or someone that you like very much. When I imagine this, I feel a great deal of tension up and down my legs, as though I am trying with all my might to hold on to my place. It's actually the opposite reaction to the one I just described, but I notice that I feel the conflict in many of the same points.

The legs develop as a result of the way they are used, both physically and psychoemotionally. Conversely, different types of leg structure seem to predispose themselves to specific styles of behavior. While there are obviously many ways that legs can be shaped and proportioned, I have noticed four basic types of leg development that characterize the extreme ways in which a person might ground and motivate himself. They are: (1) weak, underdeveloped legs; (2) massive, overmuscled legs; (3) fat, underdeveloped legs; and (4) thin, tight legs.

Weak, Underdeveloped Legs

The person with weak, underdeveloped legs may have difficulty grounding himself effectively because of the weakness and frailty of his self-support system. It will be hard for him to "stand on his own two feet," or in some instances, it can be taken quite literally that he "doesn't have a leg to stand on." As a result, he may be tentative about his self-image and position in life and dependent on others for support and confidence.

People with underdeveloped energetic charge and musculature in their legs will frequently be forced to overcompensate in other bodymind areas. Often, they will "stand their ground" with their arms, neck, jaws, eyes, or intellect to make up for the lack of strength and support in their legs.

Massive, Overmuscled Legs

Massive, overmuscled legs usually reflect a rigid personality. A person who has developed his legs in this fashion has spent a great deal of time "holding on," and is probably very good at it. The problem is, however, that it may be all he can do. As a result, he may have a difficult time with change, movement, and any form of unstructured, spontaneous activity. By overdeveloping his self-control and his ability to ground himself, this individual has, in a sense, become weighed down by his own compulsiveness and rigidity.

Fat, Underdeveloped Legs

This type of leg form will usually characterize a person who is extremely sluggish in his ability to move through the world. He may have difficulty initiating action and following through on any energetic activity. In a way, he will be like the leaden-footed person that I discussed earlier in this chapter, in that his congested way of being in the world will tend to keep him weighed down and, therefore, unable to lift himself upward and outward into his life.

Thin, Tight Legs

Thin, tight legs can usually be found on people who are go-getters. The energetic flow into these legs is intense and vital, yet it seems to flow in fits and spurts and there are often points of conflict and dis-ease at the leg joints. As a result, this person will probably move through life in a somewhat erratic and inconsistent fashion, sometimes with great flow and motivation and other times with utter clumsiness. This person usually has developed a need to mobilize himself through the world but has not fully developed the corresponding ease and fluidity that would allow him to move in an integrated and consistent fashion.

I recently conducted a Bodymind workshop during which we spent a great deal of time exploring our legs. At one point in the workshop, one woman asked me what I thought tension in the back of the legs was related to. As soon as she asked this question, many more of the group members also expressed an interest in discovering the meaning of this phenomenon, for they too experienced tightness in the backs of their legs. One of the simplest ways to discover if you are tight in this region of your bodymind is to bend over and try to touch your toes without locking or bending your knees. If you can touch your palms to the floor, you have nothing to be concerned about. If you can't touch your knees, you might want to read the next few paragraphs closely.

I decided that the best way for these people to discover the psychosomatic qualities of the backs of their legs would be for them to explore the tension themselves. So, I asked all the workshop participants to find partners and pair off. Then one member of each pair would stand with his eyes closed while his partner stood a few feet behind facing in the same direction. The partner with closed eyes was asked to fall back and let his partner catch him before he landed on the floor. You might try this exercise with a friend and see what it feels like. It is a simple "trust" exercise and is designed to allow you to get a physical sense of how you feel about falling backward and being caught by another person. When you fall back in this way, you discover that certain parts of your bodymind have difficulty letting go. I have discovered that this simple exercise usually reveals quite a bit about the way a person attempts to let go of control, how easily he lets go, and how he might actually continue to hold on long after he has seemingly let go.

After all the workshop participants had tried this exercise and thought about it for a while, we discussed our reactions to the experience. Nearly all of the group members reported that they related the sensation of "letting go" to the muscles of the backs of their legs, lower back, and neck. In addition, the feeling of letting go was frequently accompanied by a release of tension in the belly. There was a consensus that the hamstring muscles in the backs of their legs were related to self-control, a difficulty in letting go, and the fears of falling, falling over, falling in love, losing touch with reality, losing consciousness, being rejected, being abandoned, being taken advantage of, being controlled, loss of support, loss of self, and loss of life.

The reports of these workshop members concurred with my own observations, for I have come to believe that psychosomatic tension in this bodymind region, no matter what the overall leg structure, usually relates to the way that we hold on "for dear life." With the ever-changing moods, styles, tempos, and passions of our contemporary society, it is no wonder that we are all a bit afraid that the floor is sliding out from under us. In response to the accelerating motion of our human ground, we grasp tightly with our legs, forcing our hamstrings to rigidify and shorten, thereby interrupting our connection with the earth even more.

Luckily, however, the muscles of the legs seem in many cases to be extremely responsive to constructive stretching and exercising. Similarly, many people seem able to consciously relax their "foothold" with the development of a graceful and secure self-image, which is one of the aims of most psychotherapeutic processes.[14]

CHAPTER

4

PELVIS

YOUR PELVIS IS roughly the area that would be delineated on your body if you were wearing undershorts. But before I proceed to discuss the ways in which the pelvis reflects psychological history and personal style, it would be helpful once again for you to take a few minutes to examine your pelvis. You might go over to a full-length mirror and, with your clothes off, take a good look at the way in which your pelvis is shaped. Is it wide or narrow? Does it seem to be tipped backward or forward? In what ways do you feel that your pelvis brings you either pleasure or pain? Does it function well? That is, have you suffered from any physical or medical problems in this region of your bodymind, and are your anal and genital regions well functioning and vital? As you continue to look at your pelvis, move it around a bit and get a sense of whether or not it is flexible. Try to feel what muscles connect your pelvis to your legs and to your spine and back. Are these muscles strong? tight? flexible? weak? rigid? Do you like your pelvis? If so, why? If not, why not? How might you make your pelvis a more alive and pleasurable bodymind region?

The pelvis is an important region of the bodymind for a great many reasons. Structurally, it is the foundation upon which the entire upper body rests. The pelvis makes the crucial connections between the legs and feet on the one hand and the spinal cord and torso on the other. This is also the region of the body that contains the coccygeal and sacral vertebrae. These vertebrae are responsible for the nerve routes that activate the anal/sexual aspects of the bodymind and supply the energy that vitalizes and animates the legs. Because of the position of the pelvis as a major bodymind unit and its function as the hinge which mediates between the upper and lower halves of the body, its healthy and flexible functioning must be considered a necessity for a vital, free-flowing bodymind.

There is some disagreement among the various bodymind disciplines about the proper positioning of the pelvis. Ida Rolf (structural integration)[1] believes that the pelvis should be horizontal and that it should rest perpendicular to the straight line that passes from head to foot through the erect body. If the pelvis were filled out all around so that it looked like a bowl, this bowl would be horizontal and could contain liquid to the brim without any spill.

Lowen (bioenergetics),[2] on the other hand, would prefer to see the pelvis rotated slightly under, which would cause a forward tipping of the bowl. In this position, the belly protrudes somewhat, allowing the gut to remain expanded.

I personally don't feel that either of these two possible positions is "right," although together they do indicate a range of pelvic positioning that in many cases proves to be the most functional for the normal human structure. Yet, I know many people whose pelvises are tipped either farther under or farther upward than either Rolf or Lowen would consider healthy who impress me as living very full, vital lives. As with all the other bodymind adaptations, each type of pelvis positioning tends to predispose itself to a particular style of being in the world, just as, conversely, the way in which a person deals with the pelvic aspects of his life will be reflected in the way he holds and uses this vital bodymind region. Just as there are no "perfect" or "ideal" people, there aren't any "ideal" pelvises.

However, in keeping with my belief that certain bodymind styles tend to create unnecessary stress and imbalance within the organism itself, I try to look at the pelvis in terms of how it might be best situated within each unique individual so that he can approach his life from the most vital, healthy, and expansive of all possible postures. Once again, I do not compare people to some "ideal" standard. Rather, I try to explore the ways in which they themselves are creating unnecessary stress, conflict, and unconsciousness within their bodyminds and then try to work toward improving the overall psychosomatic situation.

For example, I get many complaints relating to the pelvic region from people whose pelvises are tipped either excessively forward and upward, or excessively downward and under.

Pelvis Tipped Upward

When the pelvis is tipped upward (so that the liquid would flow from the back of the bowl), causing a flattening of the lower back, there tends to be a lessening of sexual energy and focus. This pelvic position is usually associated with a holding in of sexual feelings. It is not uncommon to find that when the pelvis is situated in this position it tends to be rather trim and undeveloped. People with flat rear ends also frequently have legs that are either rigid or undeveloped, displaying a corresponding inability to stay focused or grounded in any emotional activity.

For this person, the sexual encounter tends to be just another form of challenge and achievement, as the empha-

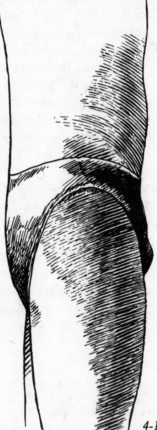

4-1. *Pelvis Tipped Upward*

sis is not on feelings, for the feelings are constricted and constrained, but rather on accomplishment or appeasement, for most of the energetic involvement comes from the head and upper body. This is not to say that the person will approach the sexual experience from an uncaring attitude, but rather that his bodymind seems to predispose him to certain aspects of the sexual encounter to the exclusion of the others.

Structurally, I have noticed that when people have their pelvises excessively tipped in this fashion, there tends to be a decrease in the amount of energy that goes into the legs, which have to do with grounding and focus, and the belly, which is concerned with feeling, and a corresponding over-development of the chest, which has to do with expressing and controlling, and the head, which is concerned with thinking and rationalizing. As a result, many of these people are prone to suffer from a variety of corresponding physical problems, including frequent leg injuries, sexual dysfunction, bladder irritability, abdominal tension, hemorrhoids, lower back pain, and tension headaches.

Pelvis Tipped Downward

At the other extreme, when the pelvis is tipped excessively under and downward (so that the liquid would flow out from the front of the bowl), causing an extreme curvature of the lower spine, there tends to be a heightening of sexual energy and sexual focus. As a result, this person will tend to be very sensual and feeling-oriented and might even lean toward being obsessed with sexual contact. However, even though this person will tend to be sexually charged, he might have difficulty with sexual release, for there just seems to be too much energy involved for him ever to be truly able to let go comfortably. I have noticed that when people have over-congested energy in their pelvis, they seek frequent sexual release but at the same time hold back against the release, for to give in to such powerful feelings would mean nothing short of letting go of all the emotions that are stored in the pelvis and belly.

Structurally, I have noticed that when the pelvis is excessively tipped in this fashion, it is often accompanied

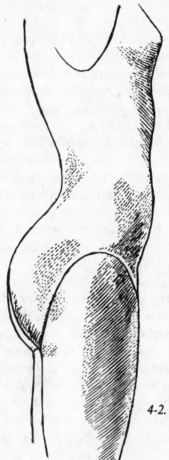

4-2. *Pelvis Tipped
Downward*

by over-developed legs, expressing a strong need for security, an expanded belly, due partly to the effect of the
tipped pelvis, expressing an abundance of internal feelings, a rigid diaphragm, expressing withheld anger, and a
tense or weak chest region, reflecting an undeveloped
ability to be self-expressive and self-assertive. The physical symptoms that seem to frequently accompany this particular bodymind posture are eliminative disorders, hem-

orrhoids, lower back pain, gastrointestinal stress, and a proneness to chest-related disorders such as asthma, chest colds, and bronchitis.

For my purposes here, I am going to separate the pelvis into two general regions: the anal and the genital.

THE ANAL REGION

The anal portion of the bodymind includes the backside, the anus, the tail end of the spine, and all the corresponding muscles and organs. In addition to being at the end of the alimentary or digestive canal and the lower section of the spinal column, this region also marks the base of what in tantric yoga is called "Kundalini energy." In order to explore fully the nature and significance of this region and also to lay the necessary foundation for the bodymind analyses to follow, I will digress for a moment to explain how the concept of Kundalini energy applies to my discussion of the ways psychological attitudes situate themselves at specific locations in the physical body and how, conversely, the physical body is shaped to accommodate psychological preference or structure. This explanation is crucial at this point, for it will not only allow me to discuss the pelvis more fully but will also help me to create the structure through which the rest of this book will evolve.

Kundalini Yoga

Kundalini yoga, which is a division of tantric yoga, has of late had a great deal of attention here in the United States. From this particular branch of yoga comes a highly structured method of self-development through careful exercises and meditation, as well as a fascinating way of viewing body/mind relationships. My own interest in Kundalini yoga began when I first realized that the Kundalini perspective on psychosomatic structure and process is in some ways remarkably similar to some of the Western approaches, such as bioenergetics, Reichian energetics, Rolfing, and chiropractic.

The central idea of Kundalini yoga is that within the interior of the spine, in a hollow region that is called the canalis centralis, is an energy conduit that the Hindus call "Sushumna." Along this conduit, from the base of the anus to the top of the head, flows the most powerful of all psychic energies, Kundalini energy. In addition, on either side of this canal are two additional energy channels, one called the "Ida," which originates on the right of the base of the spine, and the other the "Pingala," which begins on the left. These two psychic currents, which correspond to the male (Ida) and female (Pingala) life forces, are said to coil upward around the spine and the Sushumna like snakes, crisscrossing at seven important locations. Each of these seven vortexes is called a "chakra," or "energy wheel" and is viewed as a consciousness center. According to the ancient Hindu literature, each chakra is concerned with very specific aspects of human behavior and development. Since the psychosomatic nature of each chakra is related to a particular point along the spine as well as to a specific level of psychoemotional development, the Kundalini yogi's lifelong task is to develop himself in such a way as to evolve through the various chakra qualities and challenges, thereby bringing the focus of the Kundalini energy upward from the base of his spine to the top of his head.

The mindful yogi is challenged not only to activate these bodymind centers and to release their stored energy but also to keep the dual energy forces of the Ida and the Pingala in harmonious balance with each other.

Within the Kundalini system of viewing and exploring the bodymind, there are many useful metaphors that shed a great deal of light on different levels of concern and awareness in the human organism. For this reason, and because the Kundalini chakra relationships are so similar to the ones that I have discovered in my own research, as well as those that have been proposed by Westerners such as Reich and Lowen, I have decided to include several bits of information from the Kundalini system in my discussion here. Whether or not you are interested in the more esoteric Kundalini system is not relevant to my purposes in this book. What is interesting, however, is to examine the descriptions of psychosomatic unity and structure that are offered by this many-thousand-year-old discipline and compare them with the recently uncovered and popularized notions of modern-day humanistic psychology and holistic medicine. I think that you'll be surprised at the similarities.

Just what are the seven chakras and to what aspects of human development do they correspond? Although I will be answering these questions in greater detail as I proceed to explore and discuss all the related bodymind regions, I will offer a brief description of all the chakras here. The seven chakras in the ascending order that they are manifested in the human bodymind are as follows:

CHAKRA 1 Root chakra, "Muladhara." Located at the base of the spine; relates to the grand human potential, primitive energy, and basic survival needs.

CHAKRA 2 Spleen or splenic chakra, "Svadhisthana." Located at the level of the genitals; relates to sexual drives and primary interpersonal relationships.

CHAKRA 3 Navel or umbilical chakra, "Manipura." Located at the navel; relates to raw emotions, power drives, and social identification.

CHAKRA 4 Heart or cardiac chakra, "Anahata." Located over the heart; relates to feelings of affection, love, and self-expression.

CHAKRA 5 Throat or laryngeal chakra, "Vishuddha."

4-3. *The Seven Kundalini Chakras*

Located at the front of the throat; relates to thought communication, expression, and self-identification.

CHAKRA 6 Brow or frontal chakra, "Ajna." Located in the space between the eyebrows; relates to the powers of mind and heightened self-awareness.

CHAKRA 7 Crown or coronal chakra, "Sahasrara." Located on the top of the head; relates to the experience of self-realization or enlightenment.

We immediately see that each of these chakras not only corresponds to a specific region of the physical body but also relates to a particular category or quality of human behavior and development. In addition, there seems to be a progression implied in the descriptive locations of these chakras that suggests a path along which an individual might travel on his personal road to optimal bodymind health and a full realization of his human potentialities. For, according to the map offered by the body itself, on his path to self-discovery the explorer of life passes through his history and planetary roots (the feet and the legs); basic survival needs (the anus and the first chakra region); sexual drives and primary interpersonal relationships (the genitals and the second chakra region); raw emotion, power drives, and social identification (the belly, the lower back, and the third chakra region); compassion, love, and self-expression (the chest, the arms, the upper back, and the fourth chakra region); thought communication and self-identification (the throat, the neck, the jaw, and the fifth chakra region); expanded mental powers and heightened self-awareness (the face and the sixth chakra region); and on toward self-realization or enlightenment (the seventh chakra region).[3]

There are many people who feel that each ascending chakra, with its corresponding qualities of human behavior, must be unblocked and developed before the next region can be fully and fruitfully explored. In this way, the various qualities and characteristics of the seven chakras are seen, not as elements to be ignored or avoided, but rather as creative challenges to be cultivated and transformed.

This is not to say that each bodymind region cannot be studied and actualized unless it is explored in a certain order, but rather that the implied order of the chakras seems to suggest a sensible path along which to make this self-exploratory journey. Each of the chakra regions of the bodymind is said to project a specific vibration much like the vibrations that musical instruments produce, with the lowest chakra creating the deepest, densest vibration. Each ascending chakra is said to project a less dense, less deep, vibratory tone with the seventh chakra representing the seat of the highest energy vibration in ourselves.[4]

From this perspective, the lower chakra regions can be seen to serve as the foundation upon which the higher, more refined potentials rest. It also suggests that those who leave unresolved tension in the lower chakras run the risk of contaminating the more sensitive concerns and elements of the upper chakra segments.

An example of the type of problems that arise when people "skip" chakras is pointed out in the following passage by William Schutz:

> The order of the chakras is important. I've seen several people try to attain a higher chakra without going through the lower ones. On lower levels this phenomenon is very typical. A man in an encounter group is having difficulty establishing a love relation (fourth chakra) with a woman in the group. She reports that she feels some phoniness in his approach and feeling. What frequently results is that he has a sexual desire (second chakra) for her and is not acknowledging that this issue must be dealt with first. Or sometimes he has great hostility toward women (third chakra) that he is not dealing with. The order of the chakras supports the idea that in order to reach the highest levels of joy and

ecstasy, or even real affection, the sexual and aggressive feelings must be dealt with satisfactorily.[5]

Or perhaps it is your wish to develop your psychic powers more fully (sixth chakra) and you are still somewhat blocked and undeveloped in relation to personal power and self-control (third chakra). You might find, then, that your aspiration toward higher psychic awareness is due primarily to your need for power and performance. As a result, you would not be using these powers (if you were able to discover them within you) from a place of love and selflessness; instead, they would be just another tool with which you would try to promote yourself.

Now, in order to begin examining this bodymind journey, let us return to the area of the first Kundalini chakra, which, as I have already mentioned, corresponds to the anal region of the bodymind.

The first, or "Muladhara," chakra is positioned at the base of the spine and connects with the fourth sacral vertebra. It is responsible for basic survival needs and actions, and, with the corresponding anal region, is said to be the vortex around which the energies and attitudes of primitive, material concerns revolve.

When a person is tense and tight in this bodymind region, it indicates that he is overconcerned with material and survival needs. As a result, he will have difficulty giving and taking in an unrestrained fashion and may try to hoard and possess everything with which he comes in contact. Conversely, when there is vitality and flexibility in this region, it reflects an open, giving, free-flowing way of being in the world.

Before I explain this region more specifically, take a moment to close your eyes, and then tighten your anal sphincter muscles. Relax the muscles, and then do it again. This

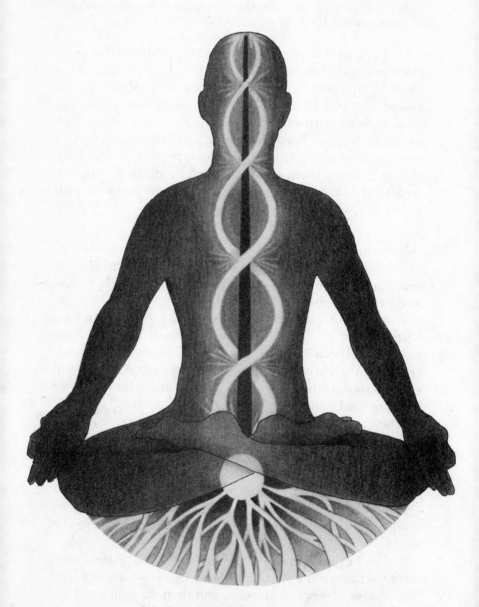

4-4. First Chakra: The Root Chakra

time, tighten the anal sphincter muscles and also be aware of the other muscles that you tighten unconsciously along with these tiny muscles. Chances are, many of you also tightened your gluteus maximus muscles (buttock muscles), your abdominal muscles, and the muscles of your pelvic diaphragm (the collection of muscles that rests along the floor of your backside and surround not only your anus but your genitals as well). In addition, I am sure that some of you also tightened the muscles in your legs, your lower back, your jaw, your forearms, and so on. Why? I have begun to observe a fascinating set of relationships that surround the use of these muscles and also underlie a great many of our character traits as well. It will probably be most helpful to discuss the physical aspects of this process first.

The anal sphincter muscles are supposed to be developed when a child is being toilet trained. Ideally, there is no need for the child to hold or strain all of the rest of the muscles of his body when he is involved in this elimination process. Yet, strangely enough, when learning to defecate, many of us don't learn how to distinguish the different muscle regions that surround our anuses. As a result, we learn to use many of the various muscles in our backsides as though they were stuck together and unable to function free of each other. When this happens, the muscles of the pelvis lose their flexibility and tone and form a band of armorlike muscular tension that chronically surrounds the entire pelvic girdle.

Many authorities feel that the undifferentiated muscular armor in the pelvic region comes from toilet training that was forced on the child too early by the controlling or insensitive parent. According to Dr. Elsworth Baker, a ten-year student and colleague of Wilhelm Reich:

> Life is further blocked by early toilet training. . . . Sphincter control is not attained until eighteen months of age so that earlier toilet training (some mothers start at four months)

requires contraction of the body musculature, especially the muscles of the thighs, buttocks, pelvic floor, as well as retraction of the pelvis and further respiratory inhibition. This is a familiar example of the armoring process. It effectively diminishes natural emotional expression, and especially the pleasurable sensations from the pelvis.[6]

So we see that because of being prematurely forced to defecate in a certain way, the child develops habit patterns in which elimination involves a contraction of the entire bodymind with exaggerated undifferentiated tightening in the abdominal (feeling) and genital (sexual) areas. This would imply that for many of us, the process of elimination, or letting go, is something that we do uncomfortably, with tense bodies, restricted breathing, and contracted pelvises. It is important to note that when we develop this unconscious habit around our elimination processes, we also unconsciously tighten and block our feelings by tensing our bellies, and our sexuality by tensing our genitals. And so, for many of us, elimination is a difficult and uncomfortable process that is unconsciously associated with bodymind tension and holding on and with an overriding inability to let go comfortably without activating an unnecessarily wide range of muscles and feelings.

The exercise of taking in, processing, and giving up is an extremely profound one. Freud suggested that this process and its related anal stage of psychological development was a highly critical and formative one in an individual's development toward healthy sexual functioning and psycho-emotional maturity. But many of us relate to our own anality in ways that suggest a difficulty in some aspect of the elimination process. As a result, we not only hold many of the muscles of this region tight and unconscious, but we correspondingly hold tight to our feelings, to our creations, and to the flow of life that regularly passes through our bodyminds in the form of energy, feelings, and thoughts.

Thus, people who have difficulty presenting themselves

in a creative, spontaneous, and flexible fashion and who have trouble allowing their feelings and actions to flow in a noncompulsive, unobstructed fashion will often reflect these existential tensions in the anal region of their body-minds. At this level, expressions such as "shit or get off the pot," "you're full of shit," and "let go of your shit" can all be taken quite literally.

Anal Blockage

There are several ways to detect blockage visually in the anal region of the pelvis. I have noticed three general patterns of anal tension and blockage that shape this region

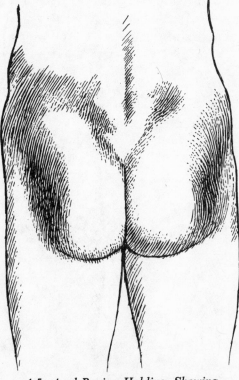

*4-5. Anal-Region Holding, Showing
Pinching In of Buttocks*

of the bodymind. These tension patterns can exist alone, or in various combinations with each other.

The first type of observable tightening and armoring in this region occurs when the buttocks (gluteus maximus muscles) are held tight and are chronically contracted. This person will look as though his backside has been pinched in from the sides. This is the typical "tight-ass" person, holding on to all his expressions and feelings. Because of the extreme tension involved in holding this psychosomatic posture, he might develop hemorrhoids and possibly lower back pain due to the overcontraction of the muscles of the anus and lower back that are connected to the buttock muscles.

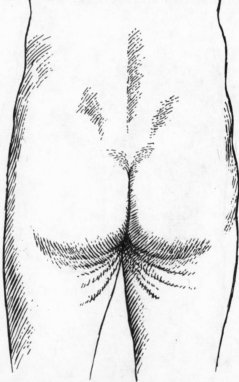

4-6. Anal-Region Holding, Showing
Pulling In and Up of Pelvic Floor

The second type of anal-region holding is focused around the muscles of the pelvic diaphragm. As I mentioned before, these are the muscles that are grouped together below the anus and along the bottom of the gluteus maximus muscles. These muscles are usually contracted in conjunction with holding in the back of the legs (hamstring muscles). In this case, the holding often has to do with controlling one's position in life in an attempt to create a secure and comfortable environment in which to function. This form of blockage also serves to restrict sexual functioning, because many of the muscles of the pelvic diaphragm, in addition to surrounding the anus, also continue up and around the genitalia. This person might have difficulty with psychoemotional giving and taking. By holding on so tightly to his backside and to his sex organs, he literally cuts himself off from many of his feelings and spontaneous interactions.

The last major type of holding in the anal region is different from the others in that the tension is generated from the regions above the backside rather than within or below it. It is also the hardest of the three types to detect by purely visual observation, since the blockage takes place within the belly and the lower back. In this instance, the feelings that live in these areas are blocked from streaming downward into the anal/genital region. This particular type of energy blockage will be explained in greater detail in the next chapter, where I will discuss the ways in which emotions flow outward through the bodymind from the belly. The person who rigidifies his anal region in this fashion frequently also suppresses his emotions, with overemphasized intellectual control. As a result, the abdominal muscles, the psoas muscle, and the muscles of the lower back (including, among others, the lumbosacral muscles and the gluteus medius muscles) will contract and tighten. Lower back pain, blocked feelings, digestive disorders, sexual dysfunction, and a backside that looks weak and undeveloped may often accompany this particular form of holding.

In all three types of anal-region armoring, there is blockage in the regions surrounding the anus. Depending on what type of control the individual is exercising over himself, the muscles to the side of, below, or above the anus will tend to become chronically attached to the anal blockage. These types of holding can be distinguished by pinched-in cheeks, a drawn-up pelvic floor, or tension in the belly and lower back. As I previously mentioned, many of us exhibit a combination of these tendencies in our bodyminds. In addition, because of improper psychomuscular development surrounding this activity, tension in this region often overflows into other areas as well.

This armoring seems to suggest that unresolved anal conflicts and unhealthy survival-level interactions will hamper further development and maturation as the life energies ascend through the bodymind. So, when tension in one region consciously or unconsciously overflows into other regions, all related areas come to be locked together by the habits and muscular armor that bind them, which in this case have to do with the ability to let go and transcend the trappings of basic material and survival-level concerns.[7]

THE GENITAL REGION

The next important region of the bodymind, also part of the pelvic segment, is the genital region. This is the area that covers the front portion of the pelvis and includes the genitals and the various muscles that surround the genitals. The Kundalini chakra that corresponds to this bodymind region is called "Svadhisthana" and is concerned with the basic interpersonal relationships that are generated by sexual interactions. Health and vitality in this area will reflect healthy sexual functioning and relating, whereas tension and conflict may be accompanied by dis-eased sexual and interpersonal activity.

Because of the nature of this region, it is very difficult to

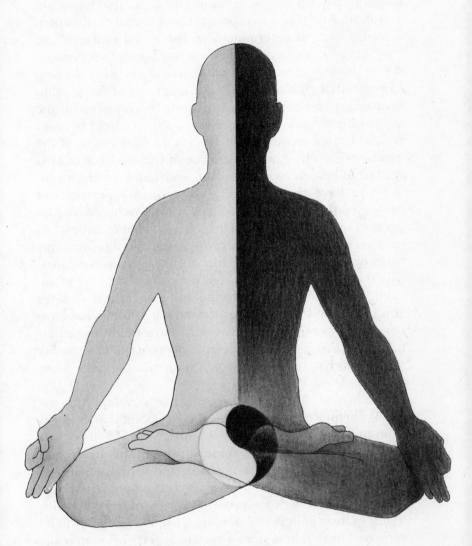

4-7. *Second Chakra: The Spleen or Splenic Chakra*

diagnose psychosomatic relationships by simple visual observation. And if there is some form of sexual dysfunction,
it is also hard to determine what the actual source of the
conflict is, since so many aspects of our bodyminds contribute to the way in which we relate to our sexuality. In fact,
I believe that an honest and valid diagnosis of the psychosomatic aspects of sexuality is entirely too complex for the
scope of this book. Therefore, I feel that it would be most
fruitful for me to pursue my bodymind exploration of the
genital region by examining some of the ways sexuality is
related to health, awareness, and bodymind development.

There have been so many contradictory perspectives
presented throughout history about the psychosomatic aspects of sexuality that it is hard to know what to believe. In
my own life I have been searching to find a conceptual way
of viewing my own sexual functioning that is consistent
with the way I have come to view the unity of my bodymind.
While simultaneously exploring my own sexual feelings
and beliefs and the different theoretical schools that have
developed in regard to this topic, I have found myself attracted to two seemingly opposite approaches to sexuality
and the bodymind: one comes from the East and the other
from the West.

The first of these perspectives is that developed by the
late Wilhelm Reich; the other is the viewpoint that emerges
from the theory and practice of tantric yoga. I will present
a brief account of both of these approaches in an attempt
to share with you ways that sexuality and sexual activity can
be understood within a holistic appreciation of the bodymind. While these two approaches are considered very different in their beliefs and practices, I think that you will be
surprised to find how similar certain aspects of them really
are.

Reich and Sexuality

Wilhelm Reich lived and practiced in the first half of the twentieth century. He received his medical and psychoanalytic training in Vienna in the early 1920s, and the major influence on his early development was Sigmund Freud. Much that Reich postulated in the twenties and thirties is just now being recognized and appreciated, and, in fact, I feel that the contributions Reich made to the understanding of the bodymind in terms of character armor and psychosomatic tension have not been matched by any other contemporary Western thinker or healer.

For Reich, sexual energy was the most sublime of all energies, and sexual freedom the highest of all aspirations. This attitude is captured in an entry that Reich made in his personal journal on March 1, 1919, the year in which he was to meet Freud: "Perhaps my own morality objects to it. However, from my own experience, and from observation of myself and others, I have become convinced that sexuality is the center around which revolves the whole of social life as well as the inner life of the individual."[8]

The healthy person, according to Reich, was the one who regularly engaged in lovingly uninhibited sexual exchange leading to a thoroughly satisfying orgasm. The unhealthy person, on the other hand, because of neurotic symptoms and rigid character traits, was unable to give himself fully to the intensity of the sexual encounter and was, as a result, unable to experience a full orgasm and a full release of sexual energy. In fact, Reich postulated that all neurotic symptoms were in some way tied in to dammed-up sexual energy.

In an attempt to understand more fully the way in which a person's sexual experiences relate to his overall bodymind state, Reich began to question his patients explicitly about their sexual activity, an action that was considered extremely radical and improper by his fellow Viennese psychiatrists. What he discovered was that nearly all his female patients did not experience orgasms regularly, and that many of his male patients also did not experience orgasms. The men may have had erections and ejaculations, but did not experience what Reich considered a true orgasm.

He further discovered that different people were able to give in to the orgastic flow in different ways, and that there seemed to be qualitatively different degrees to which the orgasm was experienced, if it was experienced at all. He called the capacity for release of bodymind energy through the sexual experience "orgastic potency," and defined it as "the capacity for surrender to the flow of biological energy without any inhibition; the capacity for complete discharge of all dammed-up sexual excitation through involuntary pleasurable contractions of the body."[9]

Reich put so much emphasis on sexuality and orgastic functioning because he felt that of all the human bioenergetic mechanisms, the orgasm was the one process that was designed to release stress and anxiety most effectively through the sexual union and its accompanying release of tension. When this accumulated charge was not released successfully from the bodymind, it began to affect the character and behavior of the individual in unhealthy ways. Reich further postulated that not only were sexual dysfunction and neurotic behavior related, but that dammed sexual energy, in fact, encouraged neurotic behavior by rigidifying the healthy flow of feelings through the bodymind. When these feelings became frozen in this fashion, they were changed into what he called "character armor." Character armor was, according to Walt Anderson, a "kind of illness in itself, a freezing of the once-spontaneous human personality into rigid patterns of behavior. Also, he [Reich] connected his theory of character to his theory of the orgasm: character was something that developed out of blocked sexuality; the fully functioning 'genital' personality had Zen-like fluidity, scarcely a character at all."[10]

In his attempt to understand fully the way in which character armor was formed and what effect it had on the individual's sexual functioning, Reich began to pay more and more attention to the various ways in which character armor seemed to be related to physical structure and vegetative functioning. At this point he turned his chair around, so that he could see his patients, and also began to shift his clinical focus from purely verbal/intellectual material to the flows and form of the physical body. When he did this, he noticed that character armor and its related neurotic behavior seemed to correspond directly to specific bodily tensions and rigidities.

His observations lead him to the dramatic discovery that all psychoemotional conflicts and blockages took up residence in the muscular tissue of the body, forming what he called "body armor." Body armor, the physical counterpart of character armor, served the function of encasing the person in his own protective muscular shell. This shell not only kept out harmful or painful stimuli but also served to limit the experience of fearful and painful emotions from within. The more armor there was, the less were the feelings able to flow through the bodymind, and the important corollary was that healthy sexual functioning lessened also. Since Reich viewed sexual functioning and "orgastic potency" as being directly indicative of the degree to which his patients were truly alive and conscious, he proposed that armoring served to impede the flow of life through the organism.

His realization that psychoemotional energy (which Freud had called "libido") seemed to have actual substance to it (he called this bioenergy "orgone") caused a dramatic change in his therapeutic procedure. For if character armor, which contributed to bodymind unhappiness, actually took up residence in the body, why not try to relieve and dissolve the armor and, therefore, the neurosis by working directly with the body? Once he began to incorporate physical manipulations and breathing exercises into his therapeutic practice, Reich found himself departing swiftly from the Freudian school of psychoanalysis, which did not identify the body as part of the therapeutic process, as well as the traditional field of psychosomatic medicine, for touching patients in this fashion was something that had been strictly forbidden.

The more Reich worked with this new mode of therapy, the more he came to believe that the only way to relieve his patients of neurosis was first to therapeutically dissolve the character and body armor that encased them, prohibiting the flow of life through their bodyminds. Then, when they were capable of uninterrupted energetic flow through their neuromuscular tissue, full sexual release was necessary. Only through the satisfying experience of full and loving union with another human being could the patient's bodymind be freed of accumulated energy, tension stress, and neurosis. In describing the ideal orgastic experience culminating in a total release of sexual energy, Reich identified four distinct and necessary stages of energetic process. They are (1) tension, (2) charge, (3) discharge, and (4) relaxation. Together these stages make up what is called the "orgasm cycle."

The full and healthy orgasm cycle is clearly explained and illustrated in the following passages from *Total Orgasm*, by Dr. Jack Rosenberg:

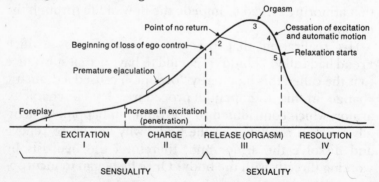

4-8. *Typical Orgasm Cycle in the Male (Rosenberg, Total Orgasm, p. 30).*

The orgasm can be divided into four significant parts, although, in reality, they all flow together. The four parts are marked by Roman numerals on the diagram [see below] and are divided in the following manner: I. *excitation*. II. continuation of the excitation, which is also the buildup of a *charge* (some people use the term plateau here). III. *release* and discharge of the buildup (the orgastic reflex). IV. *resolution* (recovery phase).

Phase I includes any form of excitation, be it looking, talking, thinking . . . anything that builds excitement is a form of foreplay. The part of the curve labeled *foreplay* is when actual touching, kissing, etc. begins. Then as excitement builds there is a sudden increase of energy that starts the curve up towards an orgasm. This may or may not be the point of penetration, but in any case it is that point where the possibility of building to an orgasm is more likely. Thus there begins the building and storage of energy (excitement). This is the charge stage. From the beginning, your movements have been directed from the head (under control of the ego). These movements can be slow, gentle and relaxed, and they can be interrupted to allow for all kinds of pleasurable things to take place, such as positioning, periods of rest, any sort of thing that feels right. If there is an interruption, it usually doesn't interfere with the course of excitation.

Now at point "1" the loss of this ego control begins. At "2," the point of no return, the tempo of your sexual movement increases, as do your compulsive body movements. At this point, voluntary control of the course of excitation is no longer possible. Body excitation becomes more and more concentrated in the genitals, and a kind of melting sensation sets in. This excitation starts the first involuntary contractions of the total musculature of the genitals and the pelvic floor. These contractions occur in waves, and the crest of the waves occur with complete forward movement of the pelvis at exhalation. In the woman, there occurs a contraction of the smooth musculature of the vagina; the more intense the orgasm, the more noticeable are the contractions. In the man, these are the contractions which start ejaculation. With each thrust the pelvis is pulled forward and upward. All the flexors (muscles) of the abdomen contract powerfully; at the same time the sacral (low back) region is completely relaxed. Some people fail to let go in their lower back region during intercourse and they experience backaches afterward. In essence they have been working against themselves. Low backaches have been attributed to "too much sex activity," when in actuality it is *not* too much sex but merely too much *holding on* that is the cause.

From the point of no return "2" until the cessation of involuntary movements "4" there is a period of heightened pleasure referred to as the orgastic peak. At "4" the excitation begins to subside and awareness and control start to come back into the body. Involuntary movement persists for a while to "5," and then relaxation takes over. Phase IV is the recovery or resolution period, a time when further stimulation to orgasm is not possible. For women this can be a period of time ranging from a matter of seconds to an hour or more; for men the recovery time is longer. Usually a man must wait for from 5 minutes to an hour or more before his orgasmic cycle can be repeated. . . .

To summarize, then, the body starts off as a "thinking" entity, getting as much pleasure as it can from what the head, or ego, decides will be pleasurable. As the movements in intercourse or stimulation continue, and as the orgastic reflex takes over, movements begin in the pelvis and you get "out of control" (out of rational control). Gradually the movement direction shifts so that the forward thrust of the pelvis is made more and more from the ground or feet. . . . There comes a point of no return, after which the movement flows from the pelvis up to the head. Then follows a corresponding letting-go of the ego, when one completely flows with the melting quality of the orgastic reflex.[11]

Once again, if this cycle is blocked or incomplete at any point in its progression, the person will not experience a full orgasm and the energetic charge will continue to animate the bodymind. Unreleased charge will continue to accumulate, thus creating even more stress and conflict.

From 1974 to 1979 I served as director of the SAGE Project, in Berkeley, California. SAGE was a project that worked in a holistic manner with men and women sixty-five years old and older to promote self-development and enhanced health. In this project, we attempted to expose a variety of older people to a number of health-promotion techniques to see if these processes could in any way be utilized by older people to revitalize their bodies, re-energize their attitudes and feelings, and stimulate their minds.[12] The creation of our project was inspired by the belief that the later years of life might very well be a perfect time for personal growth and self-reflective development. It was also our hope that if these people could find ways to improve their personal health and well-being, then we might gain some insight into the nature of many of the human-potential and health-promotion methods.

During the years that SAGE was in operation, we were met with continual success as we repeatedly discovered that older people can very definitely grow, change, and develop themselves as much as younger people.[13]

Because I work with both older people and younger people in my private practice and workshops, I have been able to observe the short-term and long-term effects of psychoe-motional holding, blockage, and armor. And I have been surprised to find that the bodymind is still quite capable of growth, change, regeneration of muscle tissue, and allevia-tion of stress even in the later years of life.

For example, during one of our SAGE sessions I led an exercise that was a modification of a bioenergetic motion designed to loosen up the pelvis. Since many older people have a great deal of tension and muscle strain in their hips, the exercise is a wonderful way to loosen them up and get them walking briskly again. The movement involves stand-ing with your feet shoulder-width apart, your hands on your hips. Very slowly, you rotate your hips in such a way as to actually form a circle with the motion of your pelvis. If this motion were done quickly, it would resemble someone swirling a hula hoop. The exercise is done ten times in both directions. All the members of the group were asked to incorporate this motion into their ongoing daily exercise routines, with instructions to pay attention to how it affected their walking and sitting.

The following week, nearly all the group members reported feeling an enormous amount of freed-up sexual energy. As they practiced the exercises each day and slowly limbered up the muscles of their pelvises and hips, sexual feelings and desires that had long since been locked away also became liberated. It was as though these feelings had gone to sleep, either from inactivity or insensitivity, and now were once again being awakened by the revitalization of the corresponding muscles and nerves.

This experience confirmed my belief that blocked energies do not disappear, even in older people, but instead remain dormant, living as memories and fantasies within rigidified muscular tissue and body armor, and that sometimes these emotional blockages can be released and uncovered through purely physical means. Once these sexual feelings had again risen to the surface, we tried to deal with their impact in our group. Among the various group members, the re-experienced sexual energy was both a welcome and an unwelcome friend, as many of the people no longer had spouses or lovers with whom they could share their rediscovered sexual passions and desires. Some of the group members felt that since they could not release their sexual feelings, they would rather not be aware of them at all, and that perhaps they had even consciously turned off their awareness of their pelvises a long time ago when they no longer felt comfortable being sexual.

It was suggested in our discussion that sexual contact

involved much more than just having intercourse or releasing tension, although these activities are desirable in and of themselves. Yet, as these older people shared their feelings and memories, it became more and more clear to me that the most important aspect of their sexual lives had come from the way that the sexual experience had allowed them to draw psychologically close to another person and, by so doing, to share the fullness of their lives within the loving embrace of the sexual union.

To summarize, Reich's clinical observations of the relationship between armoring, neurosis, and orgastic potency convinced him not only that armoring diminished the flow of sexual energy or orgone through the bodymind, thereby thwarting the completion of the full orgasm cycle, but also that the degree to which his patients had blocked and armored themselves seemed to reflect the degree to which they were fully alive and healthy and, therefore, able to experience open and mature love with another person.

Apparently, as the bodymind becomes more and more blocked, the orgasm becomes less vital, and simultaneously all feelings and interactions become somewhat limited and anesthetized. Eventually, the person loses his potential for full orgastic release as the orgasm dwindles down from a full and richly satisfying experience involving the entire bodymind to a small and faltering genital experience. Conversely, Reich discovered that when armor and blocks were removed, his patients were more able to experience full orgastic potency, thus achieving even greater release from tension, conflict, stress, and neurotic behavior.

It is important to emphasize that for Reich sexual consciousness and release suggested the highest of all possible developments in the human organism. When he spoke of sexual functioning, he was considering the entire bodymind as a holistic energetic unit; in order for the sexual self to express freedom and openness, the entire person had to be open and free.

So while the sex organs and the genital region are the primary focuses for sexual contact and relationship, the entire bodymind must be open and available if there is to be a full and loving orgastic experience.

To my mind, there are two exceptionally admirable aspects of Reich's work with human sexuality. The first can be appreciated only by understanding that, for Reich, healthy sexual functioning was an indication of the highest state of consciousness an individual could achieve. From this perspective, Reich must be commended for dealing honestly and directly with psychosomatic manifestations of sexual blockage and sexual functioning. Reich's most notable innovation in relation to his predecessors and contemporaries was his willingness to leave the domain of words and intellect and begin to work more directly with the physical as well as psychosomatic aspects of human be-ing.

Secondly, Reich must be commended for the holistic way in which he approached sexuality and its functional disorders, for as David Boadella states:

> Whereas Kinsey and Masters and Johnson split off the orgastic response from the totality of the relationship and tried to observe it as an objective measurable and quantifiable process, Reich saw the orgastic experience as inseparable from the total response system and contact-ability of a person. Disturbances in orgastic experience reflected disturbances in personality, and involved the total health of the organism in the psychosomatic sense.[14]

In a way, it is a tribute to our present level of development that Reich's view and practices have finally found fertile soil here in the United States in which to grow and evolve. Many of the most popular human-potential techniques—Gestalt therapy, encounter, bioenergetics, sensory awareness, Rolfing, the Feldenkrais method, and primal therapy—are in a way direct descendants of the Reichian approach to the bodymind, for within each of

these approaches lives a deep appreciation for the inter-
connectedness of mind, body, and emotions and a noble
attempt to further integrate them through mindful and
creative explorations and activities.[15]

This leads me to my discussion of the tantric perspective
of sexuality, which emphasizes more the spiritual aspects of
the sexual union than does the Reichian viewpoint. Correspondingly, whereas Reich felt that orgastic discharge was
the optimal culmination of the sexual embrace, tantric yoga
attempts to utilize the sexual and orgastic energies for
higher development through careful containment of the
orgasm.

Tantric Yoga and Sexuality

As I have previously mentioned, each of the yoga disciplines emphasizes a particular path to self-development
and personal evolution. Within each of these disciplines are
a variety of beliefs, practices, and rituals. Common to many
yoga paths is the belief that sexual involvement is a detriment to greater development of self and that it should, if
possible, be avoided. A celibate approach to spiritual
growth is, in fact, quite common in many of the world's
religious traditions.

Within the vast and somewhat mysterious field of tantric
yoga, however, it is believed that sexuality can be a won-
drous vehicle for increased self-awareness and heightened
consciousness. According to William Irwin Thompson,
"The Tantrics maintain that there is enormous energy
locked into sexuality, which, if released from the lower end
of the spine, can flow up the spinal column to bring divine
illumination to the brain."[16]

The student of tantric yoga trains his body and mind in
order to be able to master not only his muscles, nerves, and
feelings but his thoughts as well, until he has become able
to achieve and sustain single-pointedness in his entire

bodymind. This is not as easy at it sounds; sometimes yoga students spend their entire lifetimes working toward this goal without ever achieving it.

Once the yogi has learned to achieve mastery of self by relaxing body tension, quieting mental chatter, and releasing energetic blocks, he is ready to join with a partner whose energies and spirit complement his own in such a way that together they form a whole. This is the archtypal joining of shiva and shakti, of yang and yin, of masculine and feminine.

In the tantric lovemaking experience, which is called "Maithuna," the lovers undergo a variety of meditations and rituals before they actually make physical contact. These rituals and preparations are designed to create a strong spiritual bond between the two lovers and also to generate a mood of deep mindfulness and respect for the sexual joining which is to follow. Once the preparatory meditations have been completed, the two lovers proceed to make genital contact while maintaining the strong spiritual link that they have worked so devotedly to create.

By merging in this fashion, the "soul mates" together join bodies, hearts, and souls. This full bodymind contact allows them to evaporate their own personal limits and edges into the psychic space that they have created around and between themselves. When the lovers are united in this way, there is very little actual physical movement and no intellectual activity. Instead, the lovers are attempting to visualize

> the flow of pranic currents between them, the strongest being the point of contact between the sexual organs. Such concentration is not forced or tense, but performed in a detached, almost somnolent way.
>
> Gradually, each partner will become aware of a rising tide of pleasurable sensation, growing in intensity as psychic energy courses through the reproductive organs and the chakras.[17]

As the intensity and focus of the experience builds toward orgasm, the psychic space between the lovers continues to expand, allowing each partner the feeling of openness and godliness. In tantric yoga, the lovers do not try to achieve orgasm. Actually, if they are trying anything at all, they are trying *not* to have orgasms.

As I mentioned in my discussion of hatha yoga, there are many edges that we confront and transcend as we discover our own limits and boundaries. In hatha yoga, these edges are manifested as tension and strain; in tantric yoga these edges also are manifested as tension and strain, but there is another major edge against which both lovers are playing their bodyminds. This edge is the orgasm itself, and the lovers strive to come so close to its explosion as to experience its intensity and splendor without giving in to its consummation and termination.[18] By staying ever so close to the orgastic release and not allowing it to occur, the tantric yogi allows his energies to build and intensify, thus increasing the force and power available to him as the Kundalini energy continues to flow and illuminate his being. "Since orgasm is the peak of time, the tantric yogi hopes that by unlocking its mysteries, he will release himself from the bonds of time."[19]

So we see that in the tantric lovemaking ritual, sexual contact is viewed as a way in which two people can make intimate spiritual contact. The purpose of the sexual union is to use the joining and the orgastic passion as a way to explore and develop one's self more fully. In maithuna, both lovers are attempting to merge with their partner in such a way as to totally dissolve the material bonds that separate them and make them distinct people. With this bonding comes an increased awareness of the Kundalini energy and of its ascending path along the spine. By activating this energy, the lovers are given an opportunity to use the Kundalini energy to elevate their consciousness and to turn the sexual focus into a truly "enlightening" experience.[20]

I find this Eastern perspective fascinating because of its similarities and dissimilarities to the liberated Western view as epitomized in the work of Wilhelm Reich. As I have said, from the Reichian perspective, the bodymind is viewed as a whole. If an individual were open and un-blocked, he would potentially be able to experience sexual pleasure culminating in a full orgasm and release of sexual tension and charge. Reich recognized that people are sexu-ally as they are in general, and that in order for someone to perform differently in the sexual act he has first to be different in his entire psychoemotional system. Reich felt that the release of sexual energy through the brief ex-periencing of the orgasm, with its temporary loss of con-sciousness, was the highest spiritual achievement an indi-vidual could experience. This experience would allow the individual freedom from neurosis and would ensure a satis-fying and healthy life.

From the tantric-yoga perspective, the bodymind is also viewed as a whole. There is also recognition that if an individual is blocked and self-unconscious, he will be una-ble to experience sexuality in its fullness. As in the Rei-chian view, sexuality is appreciated as another indication of the degree to which a person is alive and aware and capable of honest, mature sharing with another individ-ual, and it is believed that to bring about a change in an individual's sexual practices, the entire bodymind must be prepared. There is also agreement within these two sys-tems that the building of sexual energy and focus, rather than its continual dissipation and unfulfilled release, is something to be achieved and enjoyed. Here the similari-ties end abruptly. Whereas Reich felt that the ultimate value of the sexual experience was in the orgastic release, the tantric yogis view the ultimate value of the sexual ex-perience as its unique ability to allow two people to merge their bodyminds in such a way as to use the edge of orgasm playfully to guide the flow of Kundalini energy upward along the spine, and by so doing to utilize this interaction for the exploration and development of higher centers and perspectives.

When I intellectually consider these approaches to sexuality, I feel drawn to the directness and clarity of Reich's appeal for sexual expressiveness and liberation as well as to the tantric view that the sexual union can, indeed, be spiritually enlightening. Yet, within my own life I have certainly struggled to arrive at an understanding of the meaning of sexuality. In a sense, it's almost as though I feel myself to be split between two generations and the different moralities that these generations represent.

On the one hand, I have grown up believing that sexuality is a private thing, something you share only with your spouse. Within this context, sexuality is not a thing to be freely discussed and casually exchanged. Related to these beliefs are a whole series of statements and attitudes regarding male-female relationships, family, and emotional stability. Within this framework, man is the provider, the aggressor, the husband. This was the way of my grandparents, who before my grandfather's death, had been happily married for fifty-nine years. In a slightly modified form, it is also the way of my parents who have been lovingly and monogamously married for more than forty years.

I have been lucky, for my parents are truly in love and share great respect for each other. I have grown up within a family that is both close and loving. For me the monogamous love/life relationship offers beauty and stability. This kind of relationship seems to help develop clarity, sensitivity, and commitment, qualities that are said to encourage the exchange of love between two people.

On the other hand, I have also grown up with a generation of men and women for whom sexuality is a changing, thrilling, playful thing. Throughout our lives, sex has been discussed openly, exchanged relatively freely and often experienced casually. Along with these attitudes and behaviors, a new morality has been struggling to emerge which places a great deal of emphasis on personal freedom, choice, independence, equality of the sexes, and open expression of feelings.

The more relaxed, casual life of a lover in this new generation offers excitement, a variety of intimate exchanges, and a relatively unbound lifestyle. Long-term commitment and stability are often sacrificed for short-term intensity and playful adventure as love and sexuality take on new shapes and meanings.

Surely there are many advantages as well as disadvantages to both of these generational preferences. Some, more traditional, spokespersons criticize the "new morality" as being irresponsible, immature, and possibly even immoral. And, on the other hand, many members of my generation feel that our parents' lifestyles reflect a more rigid, limited, and sexist frame of reference.

I think that much of the sexual uncertainty so commonplace today is due to the fact that most of us seem to be "caught" within these two lifestyle preferences. I have seen many of my single friends yearn for what they hope will be the stability and monogamy of marriage and I have heard many of my married friends fantasize about the imagined freedom and adventure of the single lifestyle. And, of course, there are those who attempt to merge these worlds —for the most part unsuccessfully. In this regard, I have watched as some of my married friends explore the limits of "open marriages," and I watch as increasing numbers of married couples become unmarried.

In addition, I also occasionally feel myself to be somewhat unsure how to relate to the actual feelings of sexuality. Having been exposed to an assortment of notions regarding sexual behavior from the media, from research into bodymind development, and from my own experiences, I sometimes wonder: Do I make love for the energetic release? for emotional support? as a way to let my wife know how deeply I feel love for her? for the spiritual encounter? for the egotistical challenge? for the opportunity for personal growth? for the physic interchange? as a means of expressing myself?

I know that at times my lovemaking experiences have taken on all of these masks and personas, and I also know that each one of them is as much "me" as the next one. I don't think it makes sense to propose that any one of these is always more "right" than the others. Rather, it is simply my intention to share with you some of the questions and probings that intrigue me regarding the subject of sexuality, and to invite you to make your own judgments.

I know that the existential conflicts I have felt regarding my own sexuality are reflected throughout my bodymind. Sometimes, I find myself wanting to open up and embrace the world; at other times I am closed, afraid of being hurt and rejected. Parts of me want to be free and independent, other parts desire security and relationship to one woman. As a result, I suppose there is an ongoing tension concerning my sexual and emotional needs that lives throughout my pelvis, belly, chest, neck, and face. Sometimes I feel as though I have internalized many of the unanswered questions of our times, and that while our culture is busy trying to find answers to these issues, my body too is struggling for clarity.

In terms of my own sexual experience and expression, however, I have discovered that the more conscious I become and the more healthy my bodymind is, the more dynamic and beautiful are the sexual feelings I experience. I have especially found that when my body is well tuned, and unblocked, it is capable of heightened sensitivity and expanded emotional experience. And when I am honest and aware, I find that my interactions with my lover are more direct, more nourishing, and more loving.

I have found that Rolfing, Feldenkrais, bioenergetics,

and yoga, to name a few, are processes that have allowed me to educate myself about the nature of my own bodymind in such a way as to put me in greater control of my own energetic flow and expression.[21] As a result, I am more able to allow my whole bodymind to feel sexual when I am engaged in lovemaking, whereas before my sexual feelings were mostly in my penis and in my fantasies. So for obvious reasons, I am especially drawn to the directness and clarity of Reich's views on unblocked sexual functioning as well as to the tantric belief that the sexual union can be a starting point for higher realms of self-development and interpersonal contact.

CHAPTER

ABDOMINAL REGION AND LOWER BACK

As I MENTIONED EARLIER in this book, the lower half of the bodymind is primarily concerned with the private, self-supportive, self-grounding aspects of the personality, while the upper portion relates to the socializing, communicating, emoting, and expressing aspects of self. As I travel upward through the psychoanatomy of the torso, emotion, self-expression, and interpersonal interactions begin to play an increasingly important role in the structuring of the bodymind. This chapter will focus on the abdominal cavity.

This major bodymind area begins at the top of the pelvis, includes the abdominal cavity, and ends at the diaphragm. It corresponds to the combined areas of the abdominal and diaphragmatic Reichian (as well as bioenergetic) segments.[1]

The abdominal cavity is the most vulnerable and unprotected region of the bodymind. If we still moved about on all fours, it would be protected from above by our back, from the sides by our flanks and limbs, and from below by the earth. But with the development of an erect posture, humankind has come to expose its tender belly to the world. Within this unprotected cavity live many of our vital organs, our guts, our feelings.

This is also the section of the body that houses the third chakra. This energy vortex, called "Manipura," emanates from the navel and connects with the spine at the eighth thoracic vertebra. It is the Kundalini center of raw and fiery power, and it is here that the rising Kundalini becomes increasingly assertive, with a passion for control and consumption.[2] As the first chakra is concerned with the give and take of primary survival needs, and the second chakra relates to sexual drives and the basic interpersonal relationships that develop from these needs, the third chakra is focused on the worlds of power, feeling, and control that earmark more complex interpersonal relationships and social development.[3]

When an individual is open and unblocked in this region, it indicates to me that he is a person who is not overly obsessed with controlling himself and everyone around him. Rather, he appreciates the importance of his feelings and respects those of others. He uses his personal power as a way to heighten his own experience without crushing others with his ambitions. On the other hand, an individual who is blocked and therefore fixated within this chakra region might lose control of his own emotions to the point where, if directed inward, they might overwhelm him with their intensity, or else, if directed outward, they might encourage him to conquer everyone and everything around him. According to Joseph Campbell, "the governing interest of anyone whose unfolding serpent power has become established on this plane is in consuming, conquering, turning all into his own substance, or forcing all to conform to his way of thought."[4]

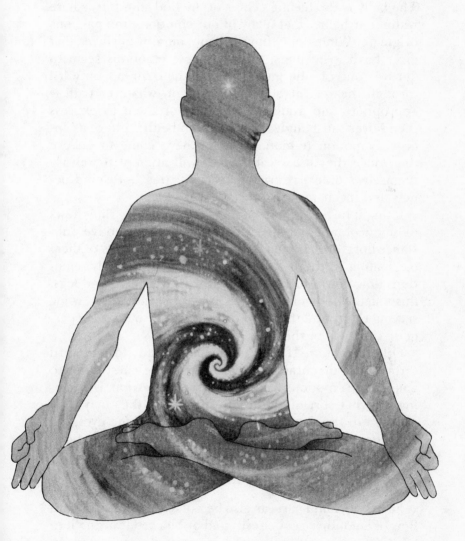

5-1. Third Chakra: The Navel or Umbilical Chakra

THE BELLY

The belly is the feeling center of the bodymind. It is here within our bellies that many of our emotions and passions originate. When something is happening in our lives that gives birth to feelings, many of these emotions seem to "grow" out of our guts and will then spread outward through the rest of our bodyminds on whatever path is appropriate and available in order for them to express themselves satisfyingly. Emotions can be thought of as energy in motion (e-motion), and I have come to believe that, once they are created, they will attempt to release themselves unless restricted by conflicting bodymind beliefs and mechanisms.

It might be helpful to imagine emotions as swirling flows of multicolored energies. These swirls of emotive substance flow throughout the bodymind, the majority of them originating in the belly, the "gut." From the belly, emotions flow downward, surging through the pelvis and legs, flushing the bodymind with sexual energy and power, while serving to ground the torso to the earth through the energetic channels of the legs.

Other emotions begin in the belly and flow upward through the diaphragm into the chest. The chest tends to amplify the emotions with love and self-assertion. Depending on what sort of emotions are in play, they may then proceed to the throat, the arms, the mouth, the eyes, the neck, or the skull, for in addition to being physically functional, these bodymind parts are also psychoemotionally functional. Each part has its own role in the expression and projection of emotions.

Each bodymind part can also be a place where the natural flow of emotions can be restricted or blocked, causing it to become stuck or twisted, and increasingly congested. In very much the same way as rocks, vegetation, and debris structure the way a river flows, emotional blocks and unexpressed feelings structure the flow of emotive energy that streams through the bodymind on its way from creation to expression. The expression of emotions follows the same general pattern as does the expression of sexual energy described in the last chapter. That is, all feelings, once initiated, must proceed through the four phases of tension, charge, discharge, and relaxation if there is to be a continual purging and self-cleansing of the emotional bodymind.[5]

For example, let's say that you find yourself in a situation that leaves you feeling angry. Since you have already developed an emotional charge, the healthiest path, from the viewpoint of energetic release, would be for you to discharge the angry feelings so that your bodymind can return to a state of relaxation and balance once again. If you don't successfully discharge this tension, it will probably tend to become stuck somewhere in your bodymind, perhaps in your belly.

Or, you might also find that you are deeply in love with someone and that these feelings have gotten all bottled up inside of you. What you would like to do is express them to the person you love, but for some reason you find this impossible. Well, this is another example of how energy might get caught unexpressed within the bodymind. When the energy becomes blocked in this fashion, the healthy tension of the original emotion begins to build and accumulate and eventually grows to be congested and, often, distorted. The longer the feeling is held from release, the more congested the particular bodymind region that is containing the emotional energy becomes.

In general, when one or more of the phases is incomplete, the emotional charge congests and becomes energetic debris that accumulates at the point of blockage, a point which in many instances is the belly. This accumulated debris is first experienced as stress and later as armor, and detracts from the bodymind's natural functioning in a way that encourages conditions of conflict and

dis-ease. In the emotional body, these conflict constellations are referred to as neuroses; in the physical body,
these dis-eases usually are manifested as points of sickness,
weakness, tension, and general ill health.

In our culture, many of us are taught either not to feel
our emotions or else, if they are felt, not to express them.
We learn that our emotions are unruly, untidy, and extremely unpredictable. Reason and "keeping a cool head"
are promoted as ways to override the potentially disruptive
qualities of emotions and passions. As a result, we deny our
feelings, withhold our emotions, and limit our expression.
Many of society's rules, and in particular, its don'ts—Don't
do this! Don't do that! Don't say that! Don't feel this!—
become the roadblocks that restrict us from freely expressing ourselves. Many of these roadblocks live in our bellies,
and many of the tensions that we feel in this bodymind
region, therefore, are due to the conflicts that exist between how we are and how we feel we are "supposed" to
be. Because our experiences, actions, and beliefs, no matter how private or personal, are to a large extent shaped by
cultural rules, many of us have, in a sense, convinced ourselves that certain feelings and actions are "good" and
"proper" and "positive" while others are "bad" or "improper" or "negative."

At times, we fool ourselves into believing that if we order
these emotions to cease with our intellect, they disappear
without a trace from our bodymind. I wish that this were
true, but evidence seems to suggest that it isn't. When an
emotion is blocked before it is fully expressed, the energetic
charge of the emotion and of the experience that gave birth
to the emotion seems to become stressfully trapped within
the part of the bodymind that corresponds to the blockage.
In many instances, this part is the gut. As a result, this
bodymind region will tend to shape and form itself around
the chronically held imploding energy and the stressful
attitudes that motivate this energetic blockage. In turn, the

blockage and armoring further hamper the natural flow of life and consciousness through the now-congested region. One of the outcomes of this type of bodymind holding is an eventual breakdown of the body's natural regenerative and rehabilitative processes,[6] which might lead to a variety of abdominal dis-eases and difficulties.

I remember lying still and nervous on my back on a massage table in Carmel, California, in January 1971. This was the day that I would be experiencing my fifth Rolfing session. Having already received sessions one, two, three, and four, I was apprehensively looking forward to this hour of structural integration. My Rolfer was Chet Wilson, a man whose slow, easygoing manner was hardly consonant with the power he wielded with his trained Rolfing fingers and knuckles.

The fifth Rolfing session deals primarily with two muscles. One is the large stomach muscle (rectus abdominus) that attaches at the ribs at their point of separation from the breast bone (5th, 6th and 7th ribs), goes over the stomach, and attaches right in the center of the pubic bone (symphysis pubis) just over the genitals. It's the muscle men beat on when they want to show how hard their stomach is. The other muscle is the psoas, or iliopsoas, a fascinating muscle. It is deep inside the body and attaches to the lower portion of the spine, crosses over the pelvis, and ends at the inside upper part of the large bone in the upper leg (lesser trochanter of the femur). It therefore connects the top part of the body to the bottom, the spine to the leg, and is very crucial for all pelvic movement, general body balance, and sexual movement.[7]

The session was extremely painful for me. The deeper Chet's hands pressed into my abdomen, the more resistance there was and the more pain I felt. I had always prided myself on my trim, tight, muscular abdomen. It had never occurred to me that my stomach was taut and firm, not because of my athletic activities, but rather because I was holding on firmly to a lifetime of feelings that I had trapped in this region of my bodymind.

As I closed my eyes and let the Rolfer's hands slowly and firmly work on these muscles, I found myself spontaneously perceiving a series of visualizations that engulfed me with their vividness. An image appeared that presented my abdomen as a totally sealed metal casket buried within the core of my body. I felt that Chet's hands were blowtorches searing their way through the outer surface of this metal locker. As the blowtorch continued to violate me with its heat and pain, I reached a point where I felt as though I could endure no more and began to lose consciousness. Just before I did, however, I visualized a tiny seam in this buried metal container that Chet's hands were working to pry open. Before long a small opening appeared in the casket, and a thousand colors, memories, and images began streaming out and across my mind's eye. Feelings of anger, rage, unhappiness, violence, tearfulness, loneliness, and sorrow all poured from my gut with the force of water rushing through a broken dam.[8] The images were so vivid, so real, and so definitely "mine" that I gave myself over to them and began to cry and shake uncontrollably there on the Rolfing table. Chet removed his hands from my belly and waited until I had released some of my long-held feelings and memories. I remember that my body's motions felt nearly orgastic, for my entire bodymind was actively engaged in uncontrolled movement and vibration. I was past the point of feeling self-conscious about my unusual behavior and continued to allow my system to, in a sense, "regurgitate" a chain of long-held toxic feelings.

After a while, my shaking and emotional outpouring quieted down and I remember feeling more relaxed than I had felt in years. Like a baby, I rested peacefully as Chet finished his now painless work on my belly.

When I left his office I felt as though a part of me had

been reborn, as though I had relieved myself of a hundred pounds of dead emotional weight. Yet, the release wasn't complete. Apparently my metal casket was a Pandora's box; for nearly six days after the session, I found myself crying, raging, laughing, and releasing piles of unfinished emotional history from my life. It was as if all my emotional defenses were no longer in place, for I found myself crying at the slightest provocation, raging at minor intimidations, and laughing fitfully for almost no reason at all. Little by little, all of these formerly withheld expressions flowed out from my bodymind, discharging themselves from my character as they were simultaneously leaving my redeveloping muscle tissue.

The other strange thing that happened after this Rolfing session was that, later that night, when I was back in my room and feeling extremely tired and worn out, I began to throw up. Now this might not sound strange to you, but it was unusual for me because I almost never throw up. In fact, I hadn't thrown up since I was ten years old and was totally seasick during a one-day deep-sea fishing adventure with my father. I literally threw my guts up all night long. It was as though my body was trying to eliminate all the toxins and poisons that had accumulated in my Davy Jones locker in the same way that my emotional system was letting go of its putrified memories and unexpressed feelings. When the ordeal ended, I recall feeling as though I had been scrubbed on the inside as thoroughly as I was about to do on the outside.[9]

Rolfing

Because of the experiences I had during and after this particular Rolfing session and the subsequent twenty treatments I have received, I have come to appreciate Rolfing as three separate processes. First, Rolfing provides a way of viewing the holistic nature of the bodymind with respect to

health and dis-ease. Second, Rolfing is a form of physical
therapy that strives to release tension and reintegrate the
body so that it can function more vitally and economically.
Last, Rolfing is a valid educational experience in that, while
you are being Rolfed, you are given an ideal opportunity
to experience yourself intimately with respect to your own
levels of tension, muscular armoring, emotional blockage,
and thresholds of pain.

For me, the least significant effect of Rolfing on my own
bodymind has to do with what it has done to change the
conditions of my musculature and connective tissue. To be
honest, I'm not really sure if more than four or five of my
twenty-five Rolfing sessions brought about any physical
change at all.

I have come to notice, after observing hundreds of
Rolfed bodies, that the people who seem to benefit the
most from the Rolfing experience are people whose bodies
are least well taken care of, and those who benefit the least
are the ones with healthy bodies to begin with. That is,
people like myself who regularly practice yoga or some
other form of physical exercise, who live a fairly healthy life,
and who are relatively young seem to experience the least
dramatic changes from the process. On the other hand,
folks whose bodies are tight, unused, unappreciated, and
poorly cared-for seem to reap the greatest and quickest
rewards from the process.

So, after twenty-five sessions, I don't really feel that I
have changed all that much as a result of the physical
manipulations.

Why, then, you must be asking yourself, would he spend
all of that time, money, and pain on something he admits
isn't doing for him what it is supposed to do?

The answer for me lies in the other two aspects of
Rolfing. First, the Rolfing experience has substantiated my
belief that the body is a whole and must be viewed and
treated as a whole if real integration is to occur. In addition,

I feel that the way Dr. Rolf has articulated the body's relationship to gravity in states of health and dis-ease has served to make me considerably more aware of the importance of a well-aligned, symmetrically balanced body structure. I have been deeply affected by these recognitions and by the realizations gained through Rolfing that to a large extent my physical body is obviously my own creation, produced from a lifetime of experiences, habits, and passions. This entire book, and especially the format I have chosen for presenting this material, are heavily owing to Ida Rolf and to all the Rolfing knuckles that have burrowed their way through my skin into my mind. In addition, my Rolfing experiences have further substantiated my belief that in order for the body to sustain change, the emotional and attitudinal sets that formed the body in the first place must also be changed. Muscular movement without consciousness doesn't seem to last. My own Rolfing observations have demonstrated the fact that the greatest changes in the physical body occur when there are corresponding changes in awareness and attitude. The problem I have with Rolfing is that it underplays the importance of these aspects of the process and highlights the entirely physical part of the experience.

For example, take a moment to think about what you would do if you were given a brand-new body right now. Chances are, you would have no conscious choice but to hold yourself within your "new" body exactly as you had held yourself within your "old" body. You would probably impose all the old habits, tensions, and imbalances immediately on your new body because you have come to develop a psychosomatic self-image that surrounds you as tightly as does your skin. The only way you could do anything different with your "new" body would be if you somehow were also able to assume a "new" way of being in this body. This new awareness, this changed self-image, comes only with an alteration in being, feeling, thinking, and believing. So, then, it would seem that unless there is a corresponding change in the habits and attitudes that create the body shape, purely physical manipulations of the body are left without a new mental structure in which to take root. For this reason, I feel that Rolfing is partly deficient as a complete bodymind process, as it does not allow people to experience themselves and the changes that are possible within their own bodyminds slowly and mindfully.

The most important aspect of my Rolfing experience, however, which was highlighted in my fifth hour, lies in the fact that during those twenty-five sessions I was given an opportunity to observe and experience many of my own thresholds for pain, emotional holding, and release of tension. As I mentioned earlier, in my description of hatha yoga, pain highlights the boundaries that exist between what we have created for ourselves as possible and what we have created as impossible. These "edges" tend to define our emotional, mental, and physical limits, and within these limits we often become trapped. As I have repeatedly suggested, the way to expand these limits is, first, to become aware of them—exploring their parameters—and then to begin to move them outward, thereby expanding our human potentialities. In yoga, this self-expansion occurs slowly and carefully. In Rolfing, the process is quick, aggressive, and can be painful. How appropriate that Rolfing is called "the Western yoga."

While being Rolfed I would usually fall into a kind of self-hypnotic trance, during which I would pay close attention to all my reactions to the Rolfing confrontation. What I discovered was fascinating. I learned that I experienced pain—that is, I hurt—in parts of my body that were tight. I also discovered that the parts of me that were tight seemed to be the regions wherein I was holding unresolved emotions and blocked feelings. Since the Rolfing pressure is relatively consistent throughout the entire process, my variations in feeling and experience were due largely to my specific thresholds for pain and discomfort; these seemed to be considerably different in different locations on my body. For example, the Rolfing of my chest and thighs was relatively painless, in fact, quite pleasurable, but at other parts like my buttocks and my jaw I felt excruciating pain. In each session I was able to fill in a bit more of my own psychosomatic body map, charting regions of tension and pain as well as the absence of such dis-ease, all leading to increased awareness of my own limits and possibilities.

As my abdominal muscles were relaxed and tension released, my experience of pain seemed to diminish, and my neurotic attachment to the memories and blockages that formed the physical tension also seemed to evaporate somewhat.

Rolfers have an explanation for this phenomenon that makes good sense to me. They say that they are not creating pain when they work, but rather, that they are uncovering the pain that chronically lives within the tissues of the bodymind. Therefore, the pain that is felt when you are being Rolfed is your own, not the Rolfer's, and you will feel as much as you've got stored in the particular tissue being confronted. These Rolfers also suggest that this pain can be relieved and, in fact, removed from the muscle and fascial tissue during the sessions, thereby rendering the post-Rolfing body free of long-held pain. This absence of tension and pain then allows the bodymind to assume a more stress-free posture, allowing for a heightened experience of pleasure and vitality. I agree with this reasoning, and it seems to be entirely consistent with the Reichian, Lowenian, Perlsian, yogic, Schutzian, and Feldenkraisian perspectives on tension, blockage, and dis-ease.[10]

Because the primary functions of the abdominal region are internal, it is often easier to read the psychosomatic state of the belly by observing it from the inside rather than the outside. That is, since tension and psychosomatic conflict are often not observable from the external shape of the belly, it is helpful to question the individual about the relative health/dis-ease of the related organs and the processes for which these organs are responsible. By exploring the degree to which the internal organs are functioning healthfully and vitally, you can discover quite a bit about the degree to which tension and psychosomatic conflict live in this bodymind region.

For example, if I am working with someone who informs me that he has a severely nervous belly that perhaps is manifested in intestinal ulcers or spastic colon, I can use this information as a key to the way in which he handles his emotions. In this case, such disease and abdominal illness usually indicate that this person is holding down a lot of emotional force which is then imploding within the walls of his gut and doing damage to his internal organs.

People who have trained themselves not to express the "hard" emotions will often overcompensate by displaying extremely gentle and fragile personality characteristics. These people usually display a quiet, sensitive style in their interpersonal behavior and will seldom engage in forceful or violent actions. When considering some of the character traits that often accompany armoring in this bodymind region, we can use expressions such as "no guts," "lot of gall," "butterflies in the stomach," "can't stomach it," "yellow belly," "vent your spleen," and "got a bellyful" quite literally.

My mother is a perfect example of the belly-holding type of person. When she was growing up, her parents taught her that it was highly improper to scream, yell, or show anger in any way. Throughout her life, she has held true to this training and has never yelled at or expressed anger toward my father, my brother, or myself. My mother has always been the epitome of kindness and sensitivity; her presence exudes warmth, patience, and understanding. She was always the woman to whom my friends would come when they needed a caring ear to talk to or a shoulder to cry on.

In her case, the feelings of anger that she sometimes feels are held and blocked in her belly, where they wreak havoc on her guts in the attempt to release themselves. It is as though these emotions, when unexpressed, grow within the belly to become wild animals, fighting to get out and free themselves from their rage. Locked in her belly, they take out their revenge on the organs at hand by imploding within her. My mother suffers badly from a nervous stomach and what is commonly called a "spastic colon."

She and I have talked frequently about her inability to let a little anger out now and then. While she agrees that it would be good for her to do so, all her habits and patterns make it hard to act out. But several months ago she called me up one evening, chuckling hysterically over the telephone. That morning, as she was cooking breakfast, she and my father began arguing about some insignificant topic. My mother's usual response is to take the passive role in an argument, swallowing all her anger. But on this morning she decided to do otherwise and without warning she flung a container of pancake batter at my father. My mother was so pleasantly shocked with her newfound ability to show anger that all she could do was laugh hysterically at my father, who was splattered with Aunt Jemima's best. My father is a pretty good sport, and after he got over the initial shock he too had a good laugh. When my mother recounted the episode to me, she said that while she could never see herself ever really hurting anyone, it did feel really good to express these feelings actively rather than allowing them to accumulate in her belly.

I believe that many of the feelings of assertion, aggression, and anger that we feel and frequently hold in our bellies are healthy and natural aspects of human functioning. These emotions become monstrous and destructive only after they have been continually blocked and twisted within the ever-congesting feeling center of the bodymind. When I was in encounter groups at Esalen I was always fascinated to discover that some of the most peaceful, quiet people, when given the permission and opportunity, usually turned out to be the most violently expressive of all.[11]

An appreciation of the constructive aspects of assertion and aggression is nicely presented by Jane Roberts in her book, *The Nature of Personal Reality, A Seth Book.*[12] To be more accurate, this passage was written by Seth, a non-physical entity who communicates to the world of mortal men through the person of Jane Roberts:

> What is usually forgotten is the real nature of aggressiveness, which in its truest sense simply means forceful action. This does not necessarily imply physical force, but instead the power of energy directed into a material action.
>
> Birth is perhaps the most forceful aggression, in your terms, of which you are capable in your system of reality. . . . In the same way, the growth of any idea into temporal realization is the result of creative aggression. It is impossible to try to erase true aggressiveness. To do so would be to obliterate life as you know it.
>
> . . . Any attempt to impair the flow of *true* aggression results in a distorted, uneven, explosive pseudo-aggression that causes wars, individual neurosis, and a great many of your problems in all areas.
>
> Normal aggressiveness flows with strong patterns of energy, giving motive power to *all* of your thoughts whether *you* consciously regard them as positive or negative, good or bad. . . . The same thrusting creative surge brings them all forth. When you consider a thought good you usually do not question it. You allow its life and follow through. Usually if you regard a thought [or action] as bad or beneath you, or if you are ashamed of it, then you try to deny it, stop its motion and hold it back. You cannot restrain energy, although you may think you can. You simply collect it, whereupon it grows, seeking its fulfillment.
>
> This will lead you to say, "Supposing I feel like killing my

boss, then, or putting poison in my husband's tea; or worse, hanging my five children on the clothesline instead of the towels? Are you saying that I should merely follow through?"

I sympathize with your predicament. The fact is that before being "assailed" by what may seem to be such terrifying unnatural ideas, you have already blocked off an endless variety of far less drastic ones, any of which you could have expressed quite safely and naturally in daily life. Your problem then is not how to deal with normal aggressiveness, but how to handle it when it has remained unexpressed, ignored, and denied over a long period of time. . . .

You will each have to discover for yourself those areas in which you strongly repress your thoughts [and emotions], for many energy blockages will be found there.[13] [Bracketed remarks added.]

I have just begun working with a woman who dramatically epitomizes another type of abdominal congestion in her bodymind. She is a fairly healthy woman in her mid-sixties who initially came to me complaining that she was not getting what she wanted from life and that she felt that all her feelings and passions were somehow locked up inside her, unable to get out.

One quick look at her body immediately confirmed this description. She had remarkably thin arms and legs, reflecting an inability to reach out and hold on to things of importance, a narrow and contracted chest, displaying difficulty with self-assertion and expression, and a thin, tight neck, reflecting conflict between mind and body, overcontrol by the intellect in her case. Yet her belly was large and distended; it looked almost as though she were pregnant. It seemed ridiculous for this oversized belly to be attached to such thin and undeveloped legs, arms, and neck. It looked to me like a life's worth of feeling and expression was trapped in her gut.

As her belly grew more and more filled with unreleased

feelings and memories, the expressive elements of her bodymind—her arms, legs, and chest—grew thinner and thinner. It was as if her bodymind were filled with beautiful flowers, but because all the water was locked in her belly, none of the flowers were nourished and they all withered while the belly continued to bulge with accumulating water. She had never learned how to "let herself out." As a result, it is quite true, her feelings and passions were literally bottled up inside her.

In the work we are doing together, I am trying to work on several levels simultaneously in order to move her bodymind to a state of greater all-round balance and harmony. For example, with specific yoga and T'ai Chi exercises, she has been strengthening and loosening the joints and muscles of her arms and legs so that energy and feeling can flow more effectively out through them.[14] She practices these exercises at home for thirty minutes each day. Gradually, she is learning to reintegrate her arms and their psychoemotional functions back into her life. When we meet each week, I usually focus our work on bioenergetic and Gestalt-type activities in order to encourage her to practice releasing many of the feelings and memories that have become chronically stuck in her gut. Each week we have been able to go a bit deeper into the fears and conflicts that are blocking her from fuller expression and fuller reward. Because her bodymind tension is deep and long-held, I am expecting that it will be several months before we begin to notice any important change either in her muscle tissue or in her emotional make-up, yet she has already begun to report greater freedom of expression and increased feelings of self-worth.

One of the wonderful things about the rapidly expanding selection of human-potential techniques and processes is that many of them are specifically designed to encourage people to free up their bodyminds and release long-held emotions. At times, purely verbal therapy does little more than create more bodymind tension. For this reason, I make use of a variety of psychoemotional exercises and activities when I am trying to allow my patients to relieve themselves of tension and bodymind conflict.

Of all the different bodymind therapies and practices, I am most impressed with Reichian therapy and bioenergetic therapy as vehicles that allow, indeed encourage, the conscious and constructive release of long-held aggressive emotions. In both these therapies, there are a number of psychoemotional exercises that get people kicking and swinging and screaming their guts out. The opportunity to abreact blocked memories and feelings and to release them in a safe therapeutic setting is a wonderful innovation over the usually passive verbal interactions of traditional psychoanalysis.

THE LOWER BACK

The abdominal region of the bodymind also includes the lower back, which is a place where many people seem to have a great deal of trouble. Abdominal tension and stress are frequently at the root of lower back pain, for as the muscles in the belly tighten and contract, they begin to tug on the muscles that surround the spine, forcing them too to become contracted and rigid. The armoring and dis-ease can accumulate until chronic pain and recurring back injuries take control of the health potentials for this region.

Most people with lower back trouble report that they first experienced difficulty with their backs as a result of some injury or back-straining activity, such as lifting heavy weights, sitting in uncomfortable furniture, or sleeping on too soft a bed. Yet it seems to me that the back disturbance does not begin at the time of the acute injury, but rather that the injury occurred because the muscles and emotions of the back had been chronically held and contracted for some time, thereby predisposing the area to the injury.

Why do so many people have tension and stress in this portion of their bodymind? I believe that the answer lies in the fact that this region, in addition to being directly connected to the feeling and power center, the belly, also acts as the mediator between the psychosomatic aspects of the top and bottom halves of the bodymind. According to Alexander Lowen, from above come feelings and pressures, such as "demands of authority, duty, guilt, and burdens both physical and psychological." From below comes "an upward force through the legs supporting the individual in his erect posture and in his standing up to the demands and burdens placed on him."[16] Feelings of sexuality, self-control, self-support, and self-stability are among the emotional forces that travel upward through the bodymind. So we see that the lower back is often stuck right in the middle of a wide variety of passions, conflicts, and psychosomatic needs. It is not surprising, then, to discover that so many people have accumulated a great deal of stress and tension in this region.

When I work with a person who complains of lower-back soreness, I try to observe his entire bodymind holistically, to detect which of the aspects of his life are in conflict in this muscle region. Then I try to verbally/intellectually resolve this conflict with the person while simultaneously using physical and psychoemotional exercises designed to train his bodymind to rid itself of the stressful tensions while simultaneously rebuilding itself in a more healthy, vital fashion.[17]

For example, I am currently working with a man who reported having lower back pain for nearly all his seventy-two years. When we first discussed his condition, he explained that the lumbosacral region of his back was always sore and tight and that it gave him quite a bit of difficulty in his daily maneuverings. Apart from the back problem, he seemed to be in very good health.

I had him run through a series of simple yoga postures

so that I could get a clearer sense of what types of stretches he was capable of and what other stretches were outside his realm of comfortable movement.[18] What we discovered was that his two tightest bodymind regions were his pelvis and his upper back. In comparison, the rest of his body was quite loose and flexible, especially for a man of his years. As we talked, it became clear that the psychosomatic aspects of his pelvis and upper back, namely, withheld sexuality and stored-up self-assertion and anger, reflected psychological limitations and blockages that he had experienced throughout his life.

The discomfort in his lower back seemed to be due to the fact that it was stuck right between these two rigid areas. All his life he had thought it was his lower back that was tight, and it startled him to discover that his lower back was relatively flexible but his upper back and pelvis needed a lot of work. The pain and soreness in his lumbosacral muscles were due to the chronic stress and conflict that were generated from above and below.

In our work together, we have been trying to loosen up the muscles of his pelvis and upper back with the aid of yoga postures and Feldenkrais exercises (Feldenkrais exercises seem to be especially effective with older people). In addition, I have been incorporating some simple bioenergetic and Gestalt techniques into our weekly meetings in order to allow him to release some of the psychoemotional material that is creating the muscular imbalance and stress. He is also on a daily exercise program that combines a variety of techniques such as yoga, T'ai Chi, and dance; these are intended to help him release and rebuild his entire bodymind, so that as his back loosens up, it won't be coerced into returning to its stressful state by a rigid and self-contractive bodymind.

We have only been working together for five weeks, but already he has reported that his back pain is nearly gone and that his pelvis and upper back feel more alive than they have felt for years. He surprised me the other day, when we began our session together, by bending over and easily touching his hands to the floor. When we began, the farthest he could reach was his knees.

I have discovered that the degree to which a person holds tension in his lower back is also often an excellent indicator of how compulsive or impulsive he is in his day-to-day activities and relationships. It seems that people who are extremely compulsive frequently have tight muscles in their lower back. Conversely, people who are extremely impulsive usually have lower back muscles that are relatively flexible. This is easily detected by asking the person to bend over toward the floor without locking or bending his knees. The compulsive person will usually be severely limited in the degree to which he allows his lower back to bend and stretch. On the other hand, the impulsive person will display a great deal of flexibility in this bodymind region. Tension in these muscles seems to reflect (as did the muscles in the backs of the legs) the degree to which an individual overstructures and overcontrols his life. The overly compulsive person will tend to be too structured, the overly impulsive person not structured enough. Once again, it seems to me that the healthiest stance would be neither of these two extremes but would lie somewhere between them. Thus, ideally, the individual would have enough strength of will to mobilize himself but enough flexibility to do it creatively, spontaneously, and with feeling.

THE DIAPHRAGM

The diaphragm is the flat, sheetlike muscle that rests below the lungs and just above the stomach, solar plexus, pancreas, liver, gall bladder, duodenum, and kidneys. Because of its unique position, its health and vitality are crucial to the full functioning of the internal organs and the lungs.[21]

I believe that the diaphragm is the gateway through which the feelings generated in the lower three chakra segments pass as they move to the upper portions of the bodymind. When this region is open and unblocked, energy flows freely and the bodymind experiences health and pleasure. When this region is tight or restricted, the result is a limitation of feelings, breathing potential, and energetic flow. Frequently, people armor this region as a personal defense against unwanted feelings. By holding these muscles tight and rigidifying the diaphragm itself, they temporarily stifle the emotions.

When seen from above, the diaphragm appears to act as a muscular lid that rests firmly over the abdominal bowl. Since the abdominal bowl is usually filled with brewing feelings, it is up to the diaphragm to control the way in which these feelings are allowed to release themselves. When the diaphragm is flexible and well functioning, emotions flow through it naturally and spontaneously. Conversely, when emotions are chronically held in the belly, the diaphragm often becomes tight and rigid. While diaphragmatic blockage serves to reduce the sensation of unwanted feelings, it also lessens the experience of pleasurable feelings and joy. According to Wilhelm Reich: "The reasons for this strong resistance against the full pulsation of the diaphragm are clear enough: the organism defends itself against the sensations of pleasure or anxiety which inevitably appear with diaphragmatic movement."[19]

Severe armoring in the diaphragmatic region is also possibly an indication that the individual is withholding severe and potentially violent rage, which has developed as a result of having held down assertive and expressive emotions for so long. When the diaphragm becomes armored in this fashion, it is not unusual to see that the section of the spine that rests behind the diaphragm has been drawn inward toward the front of the body, appearing as a lordosis in the spinal curve. When there is a great deal of psychosomatic tension in the diaphragm and in the organs that lie under-neath it, the disease symptoms that are frequently as-sociated, according to Dr. Elsworth Baker, are "nervous stomach disorders, more or less constant nausea with an inability to vomit, peptic ulcer, gall bladder disease, liver conditions and diabetes."[20]

Finally, when seen from below, the diaphragm appears to play quite an important role in the bodymind's breathing process.[21] Breathing will be discussed in greater detail in the next chapter, but for my purposes here I will mention some aspects of this intricate process. While most of us assume that the lungs are responsible for the inhalation and exhalation of air, it is, in fact, the diaphragm that con-trols this process. This interaction is nicely explained by William Schutz in the following passage:

> The mechanism of breathing involves the body from the shoulders and collar bone down to the bottom of the pelvis. Total breathing in should begin at the abdomen and in a flowing way come all the way up to the collar bone. Breath-ing out reverses this wave. Breathing in (inspiration) begins with the diaphragm, a large dome-shaped muscle under the lower ribs that divides the lungs and rib cage (thoracic cav-ity) from the abdominal cavity. As the diaphragm contracts, it pushes down on the abdominal viscera (stomach, liver, intestines), pushing them outward as far as the abdominal muscles will allow. At the same time, the contraction of the diaphragm forces the ribs upward and outward. They ex-pand from side to side, front to back, up and down, and each rib turns upward like a Venetian blind. The movement of the ribs and diaphragm expands the two elastic lungs. When the lungs are expanded, a vacuum is created in the lungs and the air from outside rushes in.[22]

This description of the breathing process not only ex-plains the central role that the diaphragm plays in the healthy inhalation and exhalation of air but also empha-sizes the need for bodymind integration and health if this process is to flow harmoniously. Since the ability to take a full, deep breath is dependent on the flexible and healthy psychosomatic interfunctioning of the belly, diaphragm, and lungs, it is crucial that these bodymind regions be open and responsive to each other's needs and capacities.[23] Once again, we see how the entire bodymind seems to be dependent on the vital functioning of all its parts, and how dis-ease or tension in one area may directly affect the structure and function of all other related areas and their corresponding personality characteristics.

CHAPTER

CHEST CAVITY

THE BODYMIND REGION that the Reichians call the thoracic segment[1] extends from the diaphragm upward to the clavicles and consists of the rib cage and its contents, the upper back, and the arms and hands. There are so many fascinating and important psychosomatic relationships within this region that I have broken it down into several categories, which I will present in two separate chapters. Here, I will discuss some of the important aspects of the chest cavity. Then in the next chapter, I will explore the relationship of the shoulders, arms, and upper back to the entire bodymind.

THE CHEST

The chest is primarily a feeling focuser, amplifier, and translator. Not only does it process the emotions that flow upward from the belly through the diaphragm but it also gives passion and interpersonal relatedness to these feelings. All the different aspects of human be-ing, such as emotions, thoughts, reactions, and expressions, mix and swirl in the chest, continually changing form and direction as they proceed from creation to expression. Because the chest is responsible for the harmonious integration of these varied bodymind aspects, it tends to shape itself in ways that reflect the style with which an individual is dealing with these elements of his life. Conversely, the way an individual relates to the expressive, passionate, interpersonal dimensions of himself will be strongly affected by the nature and structure of this bodymind region.

The Lungs

Alongside the heart, within the chest cavity, are the two lungs, which are the bodymind organs involved in the process of breathing. Their primary function is to regulate and process the inhalation and exhalation of life-supporting air. When the air is drawn into the lungs with the help of the diaphragm, the lungs expand outward in all directions, stretching all the muscles of the rib cage and belly.

In the terminology of yoga, our word *breathing* is translated as *pranayama,* and the word *air* is, roughly, *prana.* Interestingly, *prana* also means "life force." The implication of this multiple meaning is that the air we breathe contains, in addition to life-supporting oxygen, a vital force that we ingest as we inhale.[2] This pranic life force, which Reich called "orgone," circulates throughout the body, moved by the pumping action of the heart and by the interaction of the diaphragm and lungs.

In order for an individual to make full use of the life force that is available to him, therefore, it is necessary that he make full use of his breathing/living apparatus. Normally, unless we are actively moving or engaged in strenuous activity, most of us use a very small percentage of our built-in breathing potential. We are therefore only utilizing a small portion of the life force that is readily available to us. As a result, many of us are functioning at overall energy levels considerably below our capabilities.

When we breathe shallowly, for whatever reason, we not only diminish our intake of life-sustaining prana but also diminish the degree to which we are regularly stretching and vitalizing our lungs. As a result, shallow breathing tends to shrink the flexibility of the lungs and the muscles that surround them, making further deep breathing even more difficult and unlikely.

Many people breathe shallowly and quickly when they are nervous and upset, and if you were to experiment with shallow, quick breathing, you would probably notice that you would begin to feel anxious and uncomfortable. This is a good example of how certain feelings affect the body in specific ways, and how, in turn, the structure and functions of the body predispose it to certain feeling states. For example, when shallow-breathing patterns are developed as a personal defense against the experience of feeling, the muscles that surround the lungs, as well as the diaphragm, which rests below the lungs, begin to rigidify and contract, forming an inflexible band of tension around the lungs. This chronic muscular tension not only serves to further decrease the breathing capacity of the lungs but also works to encourage the state of low-grade anxiety and tension that often accompanies the shallow-breathing pattern. Shallow breathing can act as a personal defense against the experience of feeling, for to breathe is to feel; and conversely, to limit breathing is to limit feeling.

In discussing the relationship between breathing patterns and anxiety, Fritz Perls, the founder of Gestalt therapy, offers the following statements:

> Anxiety is the neurotic symptom par excellence. . . . Since therapists encounter it as the basic symptom in all patients, they have theorized about it *ad infinitum*. Birth trauma, choking by the mother's large breast, "converted" libido, inhib-

ited aggression, the death wish—all these and others have seemed to one theorizer or another to be the central phenomenon in anxiety. With respect to certain striking cases, perhaps each theory is correct, but what they have in common has been overlooked. It is a very simple psychosomatic event. *Anxiety is the experience of breathing difficulty during any blocked excitement.* It is the experience of trying to get more air into lungs immobilized by muscular constriction of the thoracic cage. . . .

Although unrestricted breathing dispels anxiety, the neurotic who suffers anxiety-states simply cannot follow the advice to exhale and inhale—that is, simply to breathe. That is precisely what he cannot do—namely, breathe—for, unaware of what he is doing and therefore uncontrollably, he maintains against his breathing a system of motor tensions, such as tightening the diaphragm against tendencies to sob or express disgust, tightening the throat against tendencies to shriek, sticking out the chest to appear substantial, holding back the aggression of the shoulders and a number of other things.[3]

As I have previously mentioned, while working with the SAGE Project, I and others experimented with a variety of growth techniques and practices in an attempt to revitalize the minds and bodies of older men and women. Among the practices that we experimented with were relaxation training, electromyograph biofeedback, deep breathing, hatha yoga, bodymind awareness exercises, massage, Feldenkrais exercises, individual counseling, meditation, T'ai Chi, music therapy, and Gestalt therapy. After the first year of practice and research we interviewed the participants about which of the techniques seemed to be most effective for each of them in the restoration of emotional energy, physical well-being, and feelings of interpersonal connectedness. The answer was almost unanimous: *deep breathing.* How remarkable that a process so simple could wield such profound power and have such possibilities for people who are more exaggeratedly blocked than many of us younger folks. My experience with these people has overwhelmingly reconfirmed my belief that the degree to which we allow the flow of life to breathe through our bodymind profoundly influences the degree to which we are in fact "alive," regardless of age.

My close friend, and former codirector of the SAGE Project, Eugenia Gerrard, recently completed a video documentary on breathing. The title of the film captures the essence of the point I am trying to make: "Show Me How You Breathe and I Will Tell You How You Live."[4]

The Heart

Of all the different bodymind parts and functions that inhabit and animate the chest region, I believe that the heart is the most fascinating and important. The Kundalini chakra located in this bodymind region is called "Anahata." It is centered directly over the heart and joins with the spine at the eighth cervical vertebra. This energy vortex is said to be primarily concerned with the experience and expression of affection and love as well as the expressive actions that are generated by these feelings.[5]

Tension in the area of the heart usually indicates a state of chronic over-self-protection. The individual who holds tension in this bodymind region attempts to encase his heart and heartfelt emotions within a protective wall of armor. The armor guards against hurt and attack but also locks away feelings of warmth and nourishment. This tension develops into muscular armor and is experienced as pain when the muscles are confronted. In addition, the left shoulder will often accommodate a protective attitude toward the heart by rotating slightly forward in a posture that suggests a guarding action.

In nearly all the Rolfings that I have observed, the Rolfees were consistently more tense and armored in the left side of the chest than the right. In addition, the experience

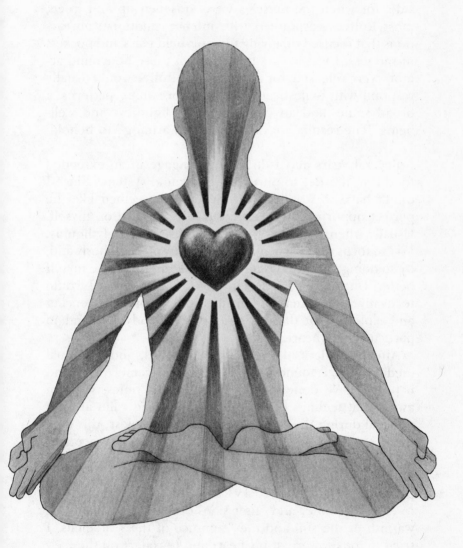

6-1. Fourth Chakra: The Heart or Cardiac Chakra

of pain and release was considerably more dramatic on this side, for when the muscles were loosened up and freed, most Rolfees responded with intense emotional abreactions that focused on giving up long-held fears and pockets of sadness. I was always moved when these bodymind armors were released, for afterward the Rolfee would usually respond with majestically improved breathing patterns, a broad smile, and an overall look of lightness and well-being. The results are indeed "heartwarming" to behold.

Several years ago I decided to engage in an extended food fast in order to purify my bodymind system.[6] Since I didn't have to work for several days, it seemed like the perfect opportunity to relax and focus inward on myself. Usually when I go on a food fast, consuming only liquids, I try to focus on a particular aspect of my physical body and, by so doing, perhaps come to know it and therefore myself better. During this particular week, I decided that I would focus my yoga asanas and my meditations on experiencing and exploring the thoracic section of my bodymind and, in particular, my heart.

After four days of yoga, no solid foods, and continual meditations, I found myself feeling extremely airy and happy. I have done extended fasts many times, so I am aware that feelings of light-headedness and calm are not unusual during this type of ordeal. Nevertheless, this time there seemed to be an extra-special sense of peace and energy. Taking advantage of this state of consciousness, I found myself a soft patch of green grass on a cliff that protruded out over the rocky California coast, and sat down to enjoy the inner and outer sides of myself. Enjoying the warmth of the sun and the fragrance of the sea smells, I tried to look inward at my heart and to reflect on the feelings that lived in my chest.

Sometimes thinking is a dead-end street, however, for when I pushed my intellect for answers, I repeatedly came up with nothing. After several hours of continual mental chatter, I finally gave up and decided not to think about the topic any more and simply to allow myself to appreciate the power of the now-setting sun. This giving up wasn't easy for me, for I have been trained that the way to solve a problem is to wrestle it to the ground with my intellect. But when trying to experience feelings, the intellect is not always the most fruitful path. Feeling a little annoyed that I hadn't profoundly answered my questions, I simply gave up. I learned a wonderful lesson about intuition and introspection at that moment, for as soon as I ceased my intellectual aggressions, my feelings and images took over and presented an answer to me in the form of a visualization.

As I sat cross-legged, staring out across the ocean and the ever-darkening sky, I clearly perceived myself as a lighthouse. My crossed legs and lower torso were the foundation and tower of the lighthouse and my neck and head were the roof of the structure. My chest was the glass-walled lens through which my heart was generating light and pure energy outward in all directions. There I sat, with the upper portion of my torso beaming out feelings of warmth and passion. Since I was at the center of this illumination, the lightlike emanations continued outward toward infinity in all directions. This light was not the same sort of stuff that comes out of GE light bulbs. Rather, it was a light composed of the feelings and appreciations that filtered up through my spine and, coming to a focus in my chest, seemed to pour out unboundedly from me.

I can't explain what I felt like as this image continued to hold me, but I knew that these feelings of "love" were not attached to any one person or thing or to any one place. Rather they seemed to be nonspecific and nonparticular feelings of goodness and happiness that I was offering to everyone and everything. It didn't matter to me at that time whether or not I got anything back for my "love." I was pleased just to be a channel through which it could flow.

I continued to sit on the cliff for several hours, until long
after the sun had gone down and the ocean waves became
fluorescent as they magically do when the moon is nearly
full. Afterward, I drove slowly back to my house, continuing to savor the richness of this image and its obvious
implications.

Later that night, I jotted down the following words:
"There is no need to fill myself up with love. I am already
filled up with love. Everyone is. The problem is that we
allow our windows to get all dirty and sooty with tension
and confusion, thereby blocking the inward and outward
view of what is already inside. Love seems to be the appreciation that we are all little lumps in the same earthly soup
which is a little lump in a larger cosmic soup. So, love is an
awareness of this beautiful energetic relationship and a
natural appreciation of the situation. It doesn't seem to be
a matter of finding love . . . it's a matter of being aware of
it. It's not a question of invention, but rather of discovery."

Before that day, I had been brainwashed, or rather
"heartwashed," into believing that love was something that
you "made," or "broke up." In addition, I had learned that
love was a commodity that could be "given" and "taken,"
as well as something that you could "fall into" and "out of"
like a hole. It had the power to "break hearts" and then
"mend them" again. It appeared to me that love was a cross
between a laser beam, a birthday present, an open man-
hole, and a trophy. Absurd.

I am not about to suggest that I know what love is or that
it is any*thing* at all. I would like to share, however, my
perception that love is probably not something you can
"have," like a possession, or something you can "make,"
like a table, or something you can lose, like a key, and that
it might be experienced as an open, clear emanation of
goodness that wells up within the bodymind and projects
out through the vortex of the heart.

I have not many times since felt as loving or as clear as

I felt on that sunny day. But while I am not always as open and radiant as I might have been during those moments, I am aware that I now have an altered image of what the "feelings" of love are, which has come to take precedence over what the "thoughts" and "attachments" of love are, and that this image is always with me. I offer it to you.

The ability to breathe prana fully and to maintain a relaxed and vital expression of love in the heart is dependent on the condition and nature of the entire bodymind. Just as the sexual experience involves the entire bodymind, being dependent as much on feelings of love and grounding as it is on sexual contact, the feeling and expression of love and life are also full bodymind experiences. As a lighthouse depends on its foundation and support for elevation and focus, so does the chest depend on the legs, the pelvis, and the abdomen for their combined qualities of grounding, self-expression, flowing emotions, and power. The lighthouse depends on its motors and gears for direction and drive; the heart relies on the mind and the senses for focus and interpersonal connection.

Love, then, is the natural feeling of aliveness that an individual feels at those rare moments when all aspects of life are in harmony within him.[7] Instead of seeing love as something that does not naturally exist and needs to be created, try to imagine that love is simply, yet profoundly, the unrestricted experience of life. Its existence is continuous, but we experience it only to the degree that we have allowed our bodyminds to be open, integrated, and balanced. Within this perspective, love is not a place to go, but rather it is a place that is here all the time, waiting to be continually rediscovered by each of us.

As a result, it would seem that the person who is most capable of being truly loving in an honest and open fashion would be the one whose bodymind is the most free of internal turmoil and conflict.[8]

Before I proceed with more specific descriptions of this bodymind region, take a few moments to explore the structure of your own chest. Is it large with highly developed muscles, or is it narrow with fragile musculature? Do you feel comfortable with the size and shape of your chest or would you rather it be built in another way? What sorts of feelings and memories do you associate with your heart and with your entire chest cavity? Now, with your hands, feel the muscles that cross your chest. Are they hard or soft to your touch?

You might also take some time to reflect on your own breathing processes. Are you a shallow breather? A deep breather? Do you breathe into your chest or into your belly when you inhale? Is it more pleasurable for you to inhale or to exhale? Have you ever had any health problems that have located themselves in this bodymind region, such as asthma, bronchitis, chest colds, heart palpitations, or emphysema? If you are a woman, are your breasts firm and full or do they perhaps sag more than you would like, because of underdeveloped pectoral muscles? And last, what aspects of your character do you associate with your chest?

In order to answer these questions, it might be helpful to put this book down and spend some time examining your chest in front of a mirror. Then you might lie down and experience your breathing patterns. It will be helpful to keep these self-evaluations in mind as I proceed with my psychosomatic descriptions.

As I have previously explained, the emotions that begin in the gut will continue on through the bodymind in an attempt to express and release themselves. If uninterrupted, many of these emotions will pass through the chest, where they will be transformed by the qualities of this area. It is here that raw and naked feelings get "dressed up," so to speak, as they prepare themselves for presentation to the world at large. In the chest, the emotions become amplified by the force and drive of the lungs, animated with the passion and liveliness of the heart, and encouraged onward by the expressive elements of the arms and face.

Unless it is blocked, the entire emotional spectrum can be seen to pass through the chest. The preponderance of the feelings that get stuck here, however, are the so-called "tender" and "soft" emotions, such as sadness, sorrow, longing, pity, depression, wanting, and heartbreak. As I previously mentioned, the left pectoral region seems to hold more protectively to these feelings than the right, and this side is usually more tender and sensitive to pain. Since this side houses the heart, it is not surprising to find that most people have developed more muscular armor around this precious muscle than in most other body regions.

While there are a multitude of ways people can develop energy blockages in this region, I have observed two general categories into which these blocks can be separated. I refer to them as chest contraction and chest expansion. For our purposes here, I will describe each of these categories in its extreme form. Once again, I wish to remind you that while very few people will fit exactly into either of these extreme descriptions, all of us fit somewhere along the continuum that they define.

CHEST CONTRACTION

Chest-contractive people have narrow, fragile chests. The pectoral muscles are often underdeveloped, permitting a minimal flow of feeling and energy through this region. In order to feel what it would be like to be psychosomatically structured this way, take a deep breath and then exhale as deeply and as fully as you can. At the end of the exhalation, stop and experience your body posture and your psychoemotional attitude. In all likelihood, your body has assumed a kind of sunken, collapsed posture, and your feelings probably range from ones of general emotional weakness to more specific constellations of in-

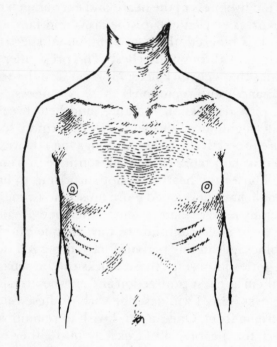

6-2. *Contracted Chest*

security and depression. The chest-contractive person will look and feel as though he is always exhaling. Muscle tension is chronically held deep and is usually associated with the blockage of proper energy flow upward from the belly and the diaphragm.

Psychoemotionally, this person will have difficulty building and sustaining an energetic charge in this passionate, life-assertive body region. His actions will be more passive than aggressive, his feelings will be prone to depression, and his actions may tend to be more motivated by a chronic sense of fear and inferiority than by a sense of confidence and self-motivation.

This person may also tend to suffer from a great many chest-centered dis-eases such as asthma, bronchitis, and chest colds and pains. By approaching the world with a deflated chest and correspondingly insufficient air and energy, this individual may have difficulty "taking it on the chest" and moving comfortably through the world of self-assertive action. As a result, this person may tend to assume the interpersonal role of "taker" more frequently than "giver." The combination of chronically held fear and self-protection, with the habitual experience of too little air and life energy, might force him into regular moods of anguish and despair. In order for this person to feel more whole, he must develop the breathing and feeling aspects of this region and learn how he might transmute the expanded heart feelings and improved respiration into attitudes of love, independence, and self-confidence.

Several years ago, I worked with a woman in her late twenties who was a perfect example, both physically and psychologically, of the chest-contractive person. Her narrow and undeveloped chest sat atop a chronically nervous belly. Her hips and legs were full and well developed. She almost looked as though she were two people; on the top a frightened, depressed little girl, and on the bottom a self-supported, independent woman. Psychologically, she complained of a lack of self-confidence, a fear of being alone, and a difficulty in "making it" out there in the world.

As a child and adolescent, she had had a very loving and mutually dependent relationship with her father that continued in modified form until her father died of cancer when she was twenty-four. Her father seemed to give her the drive and self-assertion that she needed, and in return she offered him devotion and loving dependency.

While in active relationship with her father, she felt complete and unafraid. That is, as long as Daddy was there to rely on, her psychosystem remained in a state of minimal stress. Through the years, she mostly avoided aggressive confrontations and other demanding situations because they threatened her to the core. In her relationships with other people, she usually gravitated toward lovers and friends that served to support her without asking too much in return. It is crucial to note that what was more important to her than her father in himself was the way she felt about herself in relation to her father. After his death, she floated from one man to another and from one job to another, continually trying to find that situation that would allow her to have those same warm, secure feelings again. In a sense she was searching for someone to fill the gap left by her father. The "gap," however, was in her chest and, in reality, could not be filled by anyone or anything but herself.

While another therapist might suggest that she was looking for another Daddy, I would say that she was looking for anyone, man or woman, or anything, be it a relationship or structure, that would allow her the same feelings she enjoyed and cherished while in close relation with her father.

I worked with this woman regularly for six months, incorporating a variety of processes and techniques such as Gestalt and yoga that seemed to allow her to balance her top/bottom split. In addition, I made frequent use of deep-breathing and bioenergetic exercises to encourage her to explore more fully the self-assertive, self-dynamic aspects of herself that were buried deep within her gut and chest.

The combination of physical reconditioning with emotional release and development served, in effect, to allow her to begin to create herself anew, no longer needing the types of relationships and never-satisfying conditions she had cultivated throughout her life. The empty space that her father had helped to create and fill was gradually replaced with a fully breathing pair of lungs, an open emotional channel, and the increased feelings of love and self-confidence that seem to grow from these healthily functioning bodymind organs.

When we terminated our therapeutic relationship, she

not only felt differently about herself but she also looked dramatically different. She had restructured her bodymind in such a way as to become a more fully balanced, self-supporting, independent person, with a more fully balanced set of needs and strengths. Her chest had developed and filled out, her breathing had relaxed, and her arms and face had become considerably more expressive and animated as a result of the newly increased life energy flowing through her.

CHEST EXPANSION

A person who is chest expansive tends to have a large, overdeveloped chest. This sort of psychosomatic structure encourages an overcharge of energy and excitation into this region to the detriment of some other bodymind area, usually the pelvis or legs.

To get a sense of what it feels like to be chest expansive, take a deep breath and, before you exhale, hold it for a while. While sustaining this extended inhalation, experience your bodily feeling and the corresponding psycho-emotional attitude.

When I blow up my chest in this fashion (it is partially blown up this way to begin with), I feel as though I am pumping up my aggressiveness. This "overblown" attitude is accompanied by my losing contact with the more tender aspects of myself. When I blow up my chest I feel tough, strong, and powerful. I also notice that when I hold my inhalation in this fashion, my belly tightens and my diaphragm rigidifies, thereby blocking off my contact with my gut and the feelings that live there. When I am chest expansive, the general attitude I am presenting to the world is one that says, "I'm O. K., I can take care of myself, you don't bother me." In fact, it seems to be as hard for the chest-expansive person to receive energy from other people as it is for the chest-contractive person to give it. I think that this is because before you can receive energy from other people, you first have to let down enough of your "front" to let it in, something the chest-expansive person often has difficulty with.

One of my closest friends perfectly exemplifies the chest-expansive attitude. Seymour is a man whose physical presence is powerful and impressive. His 6 feet and 2 inches of height are matched by over 200 pounds of momentum in his bodymind. His erect posture and barrel chest rest upon legs and hips that somehow seem too thin and rigid to support such a large powerful man, yet his motions are coordinated and his actions are assertive.

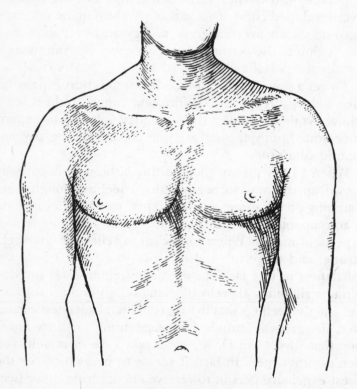

6-3. Expanded Chest

Seymour has always been a physically healthy man, only suffering occasionally from lower back pains and indigestion brought on by a little too much stress and a great deal too much dessert. He is an enterprising member of his community, a prospering and hard-working businessman, a devoted husband, and a proud father. In many ways, Seymour is the epitome of American manliness. He has no trouble expressing his feelings of power and rage. When he is angry, he yells and carries on until he has relieved himself of his emotional charge. Afterward, he usually winds up apologizing to everyone around for his loud actions and words. In many ways, Seymour is a freely expressive, fully developed human being.

Yet there is something tragic about Seymour. He never cries, he seldom allows himself to need anything from anybody, he is embarrassed at the show of soft or tender emotions . . . it is hard for him to share his true feelings. Somehow, many of Seymour's softer, more receptive qualities have gotten buried somewhere in his bodymind. As a result, they seldom come to the surface, and when they do they are usually distorted and emerge masquerading as humor, humility, or anger. I have come to be aware that the softness that lives within Seymour is hidden deep within that mighty barrel chest. As a result, his tears emerge silently, his tender passions become translated by thick muscle into power and aggression, and his heart beats wildly, yet silently, within walls of armor.

It seems to require a little extra patience to love a person like Seymour because of the wall he has put up around himself with his overdeveloped "front." With some practice, I have learned to appreciate the particular brand of kindness and love that lives within these Archie Bunker-type bodies. My friendship with Seymour, for example, has been extremely rocky at times, yet when we relax our own armors and soften up a bit, the love that is generated between us is comfortably dynamic and honest. Seymour's last name is Dychtwald. He is my father.

There are a great many people like my father who have developed their bodyminds in this fashion. Because of an overpowering need to be in control and to appear strong, the chest-expansive person overdevelops his chest and buries within it all feelings of tenderness and receptivity. In addition, the overemphasis on the upper body section usually draws a great deal of energy and focus away from the feeling and sexual centers. Because of the energy that it takes to drive such a powerful heart motor, the bodymind is forced to siphon fuel from its softer, more grounded elements.

Whereas the chest-contractive person suffers from a chronically deflated chest and a correspondingly deflated ego, the overexpanded chest is indicative of a blown-up ego. In the words of Alexander Lowen, "It reminds one of the fable of the frog who attempted to blow himself up to the size of a bull."[9] While the chest-contractive person will tend to suffer from depression and anguish because of his undercharged thoracic region, the chest-expansive person "will suffer from problems such as chronic anxiousness, hypertension, high blood pressure, and a possible inclination toward tuberculosis and heart problems."[10]

Neither chest contraction nor chest expansion defines the healthiest of all chest attitudes. Rather, it is the balance between these two exaggerations that describes the most vital and loving of all possibilities. Just as a breath is made up of an inhalation as well as an exhalation, and loving relationships are built on the ability to give as well as receive, true human creativity lies in the ability to experience the world anew each instant, to have each breath begin fresh, and to express freely and openly each passion of the bodymind. In the unrestricted individual, the balance of soft and hard, in and out, giving and receiving, expansion and contraction, defines the power and beauty of the thoracic region of the bodymind.[11]

CHAPTER

SHOULDERS AND ARMS

THE SHOULDERS, arms, hands, and upper back are primarily involved with the "doing" and "expressing" aspects of one's character. Through observing their form and function, we can learn quite a bit about the way a person handles himself in the world.

THE SHOULDERS

The shoulders are intimately connected with the chest cavity, for they not only lie across the top of the rib cage but also extend over the front of the chest, where they connect to the sternum, and down the back, where they join with the scapulae (shoulder blades). From this position, the shoulders have the responsibility of mediating between the emotional powers of the torso and the expressive elements of the arms and hands.

Once again, it would be helpful if you put this book down and took a look at yourself in a mirror. This time, pay particular attention to your shoulders. Do they seem

very well developed to you, or are they narrow and underdeveloped? Are your shoulder muscles flexible and loose,
or do they feel tight and rigid? Is there a difference between your right shoulder and your left? Do your shoulders bow forward or are they arched backward? Now,
move your shoulders around and get a sense for the
range of movement that is possible. As you flex your
shoulders, watch what happens to the surrounding bodymind regions. Try to feel all the ways that your shoulders
are connected to your arms, your chest, your diaphragm,
your belly, your pelvis, your legs and feet. Are they fully
connected? If not, where is the connection interrupted?
Now, using your shoulders, allow yourself to assume a variety of emotional attitudes such as happy, afraid, angry,
sad, tired, depressed, exuberant, overburdened, proud,
egomaniacal, and humble. As you assume each of these
psychological postures, pay attention to what information
the positioning of your shoulders projects that reveals
this attitude. When you have finished acting out these various attitudes, let your shoulders resume their natural position, and then try to get a sense of what aspects of your
character or your emotional history are revealed in the
habitual position of your shoulders.

Compared with many of the other bodymind regions that
we have discussed, the shoulders are easy to read because
they can assume a variety of readily noticeable shapes and
positions. When I examine a person's shoulders, I try to
imagine what sort of emotional experience the person is
involved in, or has been through, for the shoulders to be
positioned as they are. The assumption in this type of bodymind reading is that the person has, in fact, been involved
in such an experience, or experiences, and has built a segment of his everyday character around the critical charge of
this experience.

For example, perhaps when you were very young you
were shocked or frightened. Your shoulders flew up and

your spine tingled, much the same way as your pet cat responds by arching his back when he feels threatened. Normally, when we are frightened, the immediate threat eventually resolves itself to our personal satisfaction and we eventually allow ourselves to relax and resume an unfrightened bodymind posture.

Yet in some instances people never fully resolve their fears, and their shoulders remain in an arched and rigid position long after the immediate fear has passed. When this happens, we say that the person has internalized the fear and that the experience of fright has been locked into the structure of the total bodymind and become a kind of "frozen history." At this point the natural growth of the bodymind becomes slightly distorted and begins to shape itself around the frightened posture and its corresponding tensions. Eventually, the "frozen history" becomes fully integrated into the character and body structure of the individual.

David Boadella explains the way frozen history affects character structure in this passage from *Wilhelm Reich: The Evolution of His Work:*

> A basic conflict which a person experienced at a certain stage in his life left its trace in his character in the form of a defensive rigidity of attitude, behaviour and expression. The character-rigidity bound up the emotional charge of the original conflict, and gave protection against the stormy emotions aroused at the time. If now, the character rigidity could be interpreted and dissolved, the frozen emotion could flow again. . . . Emotion was bound up in the character-formation, and no full emotional release or psychoanalytic cure would be possible while the original character-formation retained its defensive function of armouring the patient against strong feelings.[1]

This type of emotional holding and blocking is reflected in the body structure also, and tends especially to affect the way we hold our shoulders. There are a variety of common "frozen histories" that seem regularly to get stuck in the shoulders, many of them focused around the way the person is relating to the demands and pressures of his life. Quite literally, the shape and form of this bodymind region reveals the manner in which this person is "shouldering his responsibilities."

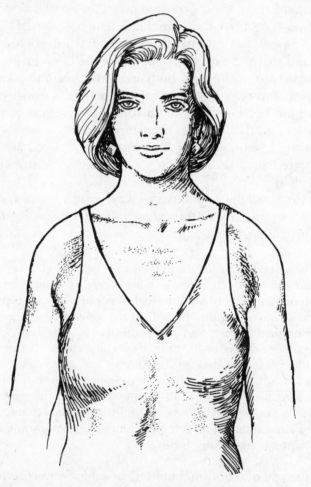

7-1. Bowed, Rounded Shoulders

Bowed, Rounded Shoulders

Bowed, rounded shoulders convey the message that the person sees himself as having the weight of the whole world on his shoulders. People with bowed shoulders seem to take on more responsibilities than they are built to handle. As a result, the stance they present to the world is one of being overburdened by life itself.

Raised Shoulders

Shoulders that are raised considerably higher than they should naturally be indicate an attitude of fear. As I

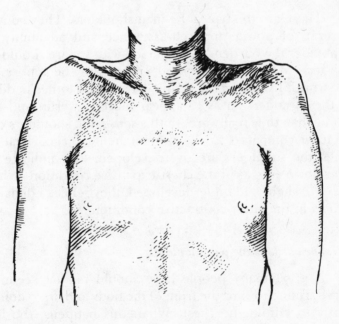

7-2. Raised Shoulders

mentioned earlier, we tend to raise our shoulders up to-ward our ears when we are frightened. When the fear is discharged, the shoulders relax and return to their normal resting position. If we are unable to release this fear, how-ever, our shoulders may remain up, locking us into a frozen state of chronic fear. In extreme cases, the individual with severely raised shoulders will look something like a turtle that is trying to retract its head into its protective shell. Since the original object of the fear is usually long since gone, the person will tend to project his now-internalized fear irrationally onto new objects and situations. This type of bodymind posture often corresponds to a paranoid state of mind.

Square Shoulders

These are the typical he-man shoulders. They convey a sense of power and self-assurance and an ability to "shoulder the burden." The person with square shoulders will tend to be very concerned with the way he appears to the world. In fact, many people have their clothes padded at the shoulders so as to appear more powerful and dy-namic than they really are. In this sense, the shoulders can even be compared to the development of ego. That is, when the shoulders are overdeveloped, they indicate an overblown ego, as in the chest-expansive condition. When they are slight and underdeveloped, they reflect a deflated ego as in the chest-contractive condition.

Forward, Hunched Shoulders

A great many people have shoulders that seem to curve around toward the front of the body and, in so doing, partly to enfold the chest. When this happens, the left shoulder is usually rotated more forward than the right. Forward shoulders usually reflect a chronic attitude of self-

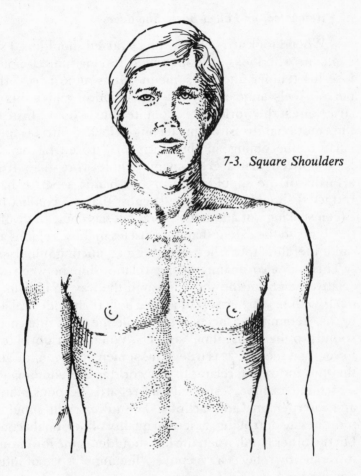

7-3. *Square Shoulders*

protection and a fear of being hurt. The person may see himself as being highly vulnerable and tender and attempts to protect his chest and heart by drawing his shoulders and arms forward. When the shoulders are rotated in this fashion, however, the muscles of the chest tighten and contract, thereby causing them to be even more vulnerable and sensitive. The forward shoulders and contracted chest are frequently accompanied by shallow breathing and emotional holding in the belly and diaphragm.

Retracted, or Pulled-Back, Shoulders

When I look at a person with retracted shoulders, I see someone who looks as though he is forcing himself not to lose his temper and hit someone. It is almost as if this person feels annoyed by his life situation and wants to strike out at the world but isn't quite able to do so. Instead, the emotional thrust of this feeling is locked into his musculature, becoming another form of "frozen history." I have noticed that a great many people who suffer from arthritis of the shoulders, arms, or hands seem to have retracted shoulders. It would suggest that the conflict between striking out and not striking out has come to involve the joints to the extent that the muscles in these regions are quite literally "torn" between these conflicting impulses.[2]

There is also an interesting relationship between the relative height of the shoulders and the way an individual deals with his or her sexual role. The left shoulder relates to the "feminine" aspects of self while the right side corresponds to the "masculine" aspects. When the right side is lower than the left, as is true of most men, it often indicates that this individual relates to the world in a predominantly masculine fashion, especially as regards responsibilities and interpersonal interactions. The lower right shoulder indicates a controlling, assertive quality of personal action. On the other hand, when the left shoulder is the lower one, it frequently reflects a receptive, "feminine" style of interpersonal motion.[3]

THE ARMS AND HANDS

Unrestricted emotions and energy flow through the chest and upward into the shoulders and arms, and through the neck into the face. The arms and hands provide the channels through which a great many highly functional emotions are expressed; among others they are able to transmit

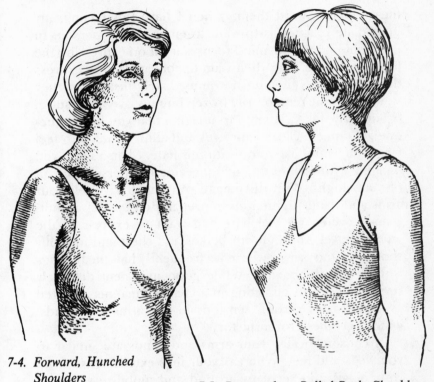

7-4. *Forward, Hunched*
Shoulders

7-5. *Retracted, or Pulled-Back, Shoulders*

and generate such actions as hitting, stroking, striking, grasping, holding, taking, giving, reaching out, manipulating, feeling, self-protecting, and self-extending.

For example, think of someone whom you love very deeply. Allow yourself to really get into feeling this love throughout your bodymind. As the streamings of this emotion continue to build up charge, close your eyes and somatically explore where this love wants to go.

When I feel love in my body toward someone, in addition to feeling warmth and attraction in my pelvis, I notice that my hands and arms begin to tingle, an indication of the tiny expansions and contractions that are beginning to beckon the feelings toward them. When I have this feeling, my immediate reaction is to want to embrace this person. In this fashion, my bodymind focuses itself on expressing the feelings of love. But when I am unable actually to express these emotions, they do not immediately disappear; they simply become temporarily frozen into my overall posture.

Similarly, take a minute to imagine that you hate someone very much. Close your eyes and allow yourself to feel what you would like to do with this hate. Chances are, you imagined yourself hitting or squeezing this person with all of your might. With this image you might have felt your arms and hands tighten up in preparation for the assault. Usually, when we feel hate and want to express it, the energy travels through our bellies and chest and into our shoulders and arms—where we frequently halt the feelings with "good judgment." While good judgment definitely serves to keep us all acting in a civilized manner, it often as well creates chronic tensions in our arms and hands, which become "frozen history."

Psychosomatically, your arms and hands are similar to your legs and feet. Whereas your legs extend down from your pelvis and serve to ground and mobilize you with respect to the earth and its gravitational pull, your arms radiate out from your heart and serve to "ground" you with respect to the world of people and things. They communicate by their motions, actions, and functions the feelings of your bodymind to other people. Your arms can even be thought of as probes that extend out into the world not only from your chest, but from your legs, pelvis, belly, and neck and head as well: they communicate a great deal of information inward to your bodymind about what is going on outside you.

Like your legs, your arms consist of joints and sections through which a variety of energies and feelings can flow. They, too, are psychosomatic crossroads, registering the flow of energy by the degree of vitality or dis-ease of the limb and its ability to serve your entire organism. As I mentioned in my discussion of the legs, the relative flexibility and grace of your joints determine and reflect the way you move in the world. Therefore the grace in your arms would correspond to the way you move through the world of interpersonal relationships and the give-and-take type of interactions.

Oscar Ichazo, founder of the Arica school of human development, describes the arms in this fashion: The upper arms "reflect our strength." The elbows reflect the "ease or awkwardness . . . with which we move through the world." The forearms "are the means we use," and the hands "are used for giving and taking, for reaching out for goals."[4]

Healthy, unrestricted arms are strong yet flexible, powerful yet gentle, able to reach and hold as well as withdraw and refuse, able to give as well as take, able to stroke as well as slap. Once again, it seems that energetic vitality in the arms and hands is dependent on the organism's ability to express freely an entire range of feelings and actions. As with legs, there are four primary ways in which energy imbalance is embodied in the arms: (1) weak, underdeveloped arms; (2) massive, overmuscled arms; (3) fat, underdeveloped arms; and (4) thin, tight arms.

Weak, Underdeveloped Arms

Weakness in the arms is usually related to a holding of energy and expression in the chest or belly and frequently at the shoulders. The person complains of feelings of weakness and impotence in his arms and, correspondingly, shows a lack of ability to reach out and take hold of his life. These feelings are often accompanied by cold or clammy hands and a sense of powerlessness in one's relationships to people and things. According to Wilhelm Reich, "The lives of such patients are characterized by a general lack of initiative."[5]

Massive, Overmuscled Arms

Massive or overdeveloped musculature in the arms usually corresponds to a lack of grace or sensitivity in an individual's means of expression and contact. As a result, he will tend to relate to people in an insensitive way, treating them as "objects." Such relationships will suffer from a lack of honest contact and direct communication. This person will resort to brute force in an attempt to grasp and hold on to what he wants. In addition, his movements will be somewhat forceful and awkward, reflecting the difficulty he has with gentle motion and interaction.

Thin, Tight Arms

Rigid muscular development of the arms reflects a kind of grasping, clawing, clutching quality about a person's attitudes. Energetic flow and motion through the arms, while coordinated and capable, are often inconsistent and spastic. Although the person is able to reach out and make contact, he has difficulty holding on to anything for extended periods of time. He may also have trouble keeping his attention and expressions focused. The conflicts that animate his arms live predominantly in the joints and hands and manifest as injuries, strains, twists, tensions, and other conditions related to disjointed energy.

Fat, Underdeveloped Arms

As with the legs, arms that are extremely fat and undeveloped reflect a deadness or sluggishness of action. The person who has developed himself in this fashion will have difficulty initiating action and sustaining energy throughout an activity, for he is so overladen with his own weight and emotional inertia that he quite literally buries himself within his own body. When this person does reach out, the expression tends to be overdramatic and clumsy because of his lack of precision and energetic fluidity in his bodymind region.[6],[7]

Some time ago I was leading a small encounter/Gestalt session in Berkeley, California, and was given an opportunity to observe a situation that clearly exemplified the psychosomatic nature of the arms.

One of the women in the group complained that she frequently felt extremely cold in her arms and legs. Physically, she was a very beautiful woman, looking much younger than her thirty-five years. Her body was thin, with a slightly distended belly, expressing congested feelings, a slightly contracted chest, indicative of difficulty with self-assertion, and narrow and weak arms and legs that seemed to hang disjointedly off her shoulders and hips. In addition, her breathing was somewhat shallow. She appeared to be very bright and a bit over-self-conscious.

She explained that her condition had been diagnosed by a physician as "Raynaud's disease," which is manifest in a "constriction of the blood vessels causing impaired circulation in the hands, feet, ears, and nose. The hands are affected most often. They may become pallid, numb and purplish."[8] In order to seek a cure for her "purely physical" symptoms, she had been to see a variety of health practitioners and therapists, who had suggested that she change her nutritional habits, meditate, do yoga, practice biofeedback training, and try a variety of other methods and techniques. All these methods had apparently helped her to become more relaxed and self-aware, but none of them had relieved her of the Raynaud's symptoms.

When she shared her problem with the group, my immediate line of exploration was motivated by my belief that the arms have primarily to do with interpersonal relationships. So I had her move around the group, confronting each member. She was instructed to position herself as far away from the person as was necessary in order for her hands not to feel cold. One by one, she faced each group member, placing herself at a distance that allowed her to feel physically comfortable. The interesting result of this simple exercise was that she located herself at different distances from each member. With this exercise, her identification of necessary personal space was immediately translated from the conscious/unconscious realm into the visible/physical domain.[9] As she got more involved in the experiment, I asked her to verbalize her feelings as she confronted each group member.

When she faced people with whom she felt interpersonally comfortable, her hands were warm and she felt relaxed. But when she confronted members of the group with whom she felt uncertain, she grew tense, her shoulders tightened, her breathing shallowed, and her hands grew cold. This simple exercise made it immediately clear that her Raynaud's disease was acting like a meter or scale that kept her informed about the degree to which she was comfortable or uncomfortable in making contact with another person. In general, her hands were colder when she confronted men than women, and coldest when facing men to whom she felt attracted and, therefore, vulnerable.

After she became more able to identify this psychosomatic process, she began to verbalize what was taking place inside her when involved in these Raynaud's-producing confrontations. Apparently she was extremely afraid of being rejected, especially by men that she was attracted to. The fear of the uncertain confrontation forced her to retreat from the fullness of her bodymind and take refuge at her core. As a result, the peripheral sections of her bodymind were left abandoned, unattached to her energetic flow—cold.

I then had her face the people in the group who were most threatening to her. She was allowed, once again, to assume a position in the room that allowed her comfortable "breathing room," as it were, from this person. As she began each confrontation, she moved to the farthest point that the room would allow away from her partner. She reported that if the walls had not been there, she would have moved farther still.

I asked her to pay attention to her own feelings as she faced the person. She was told to pay attention to the temperature of her hands and to move slowly toward her partner, in a way that did not force her to contract all of her energy. As she did, I monitored her breathing and pelvic tension with my eyes, reminding her to stay relaxed and breathe whenever she interrupted the flow in these regions. By being tuned in to the places in her core that held her contracted, she was apparently more able to sustain energetic charge and warmth in her arms and hands. What she discovered was that if she went slowly and mindfully, she was able to get rather close to the person without feeling nervous or cold-handed.

After this exercise, we shared the observation that her Raynaud's disease seemed to be directly related to her difficulty in reaching out to other people, especially people who had the power to reject her, something she was very much afraid of. Along with this realization came the obvious suggestion that what she needed to do was to practice using her arms and hands and the psychosomatic functions that animate them in a more expansive fashion than she had been. By extending herself out into her peripheral limbs, she might begin to generate more life and warmth into them, thereby remedying her Raynaud problem.

This is a fine example of how the bodymind, in discovering its own imbalances and weaknesses, simultaneously points the way to appropriate remedies and self-correctional advice. The concept is simple: If there is a part of you that is underdeveloped, unconscious, and weak, make it stronger. As I have suggested, I feel that the best way to work toward bodymind change is to approach the change process from its physical *and* emotional aspects. So, if a part of your bodymind is weak, you need to strengthen it by fortifying the weak physical regions that house this part of you with appropriate physical or psychophysical exercises and by strengthening or developing the correspondingly weak psychological or emotional aspects with the help of appropriate therapy, guidance, self-reflection, or psychoemotional techniques.

Or, if a part of you is overdeveloped or overcongested, allow it to become more receptive, softer, more graceful with appropriate remedial activities. If there is a part of your bodymind that is physically unwell, begin paying close attention to what aspects of your life are in conflict that correspond to the area of disease. When you have identified the conflicts, you must then begin to sort them out and resolve them both physically and psychologically before your bodymind can resume its most natural condition of health and vitality.

In addition to being psychosomatically related to a variety of emotional needs and functions, the arms and hands are also highly expressive channels for nonverbal communication. In fact, in many instances the statements of the hands seem to be even more honest and direct than those of the mouth. During my Gestalt therapy[10] training, I was continually reminded to pay close attention to the hands, for it was believed that the patient's true emotions would be expressed through his physical actions, whereas his words would usually only be reflections of what he "thought" he was feeling.

The problem is that most of us, being so intellectually oriented, only pay direct attention to what a person is saying with words and frequently miss the true feelings that they are projecting with their hands, shoulders, and eyes. This point is nicely illustrated with an example from *Body Language,* by Julius Fast, a book that is concerned with identifying some of the ways that we communicate non-verbally.

> Touching or fondling in itself can be a potent signal . . . or a plea for understanding. Take the case of Aunt Grace. This old woman had become the center of a family discussion. Some of the family felt she would be better off in a pleasant and well-run nursing home nearby where she'd not only have people to take care of her but would also have plenty of companionship.
>
> The rest of the family felt that this was tantamount to putting Aunt Grace "away." She had a generous income and a lovely apartment, and she could still do very well for herself. Why shouldn't she live where she was, enjoying her independence and her freedom?
>
> Aunt Grace herself was no great help in the discussion. She sat in the middle of the family group, fondling her necklace and nodding, picking up a small alabaster paper-weight and caressing it, running one hand along the velvet of the couch, then feeling the wooden carving.
>
> "Whatever the family decided," she said gently. "I don't want to be a problem to anyone."
>
> The family couldn't decide, and kept discussing the problem, while Aunt Grace kept fondling all the objects within reach.
>
> Until finally the family got the message. It was a pretty obvious message too. It was just a wonder no one had gotten it sooner. Aunt Grace had been a fondler ever since she had begun living alone. She touched and caressed everything within reach. All the family knew it, but it wasn't until that moment that, one by one, they all became aware of what her fondling was saying. She was telling them in

body language, "I am lonely. I am starved for companion-
ship. Help me."

Aunt Grace was taken to live with a niece and nephew,
where she became a different woman.

Like Aunt Grace, we all, in one way or another, send our
little messages out to the world.[11]

THE UPPER BACK

The upper back corresponds to the section of the spine that
houses the twelve thoracic or dorsal vertebrae. This part of
the body is actually contained within the shoulder girdle,
which extends downward to the bottom of the shoulder
blades. Yet since most of us think of the upper back as
being separate from the shoulders, I have chosen to present them in this fashion.

During the years I have been studying the bodymind, I
have been fascinated by the ways that different disciplines,
such as Reichian energetics, bioenergetics, and Gestalt,
correlate the different aspects of the human organism.
Often there is disagreement among the different approaches over specific psychosomatic interpretations and
analyses. The muscles that surround the thoracic region of
the spine, however, have been described and diagnosed
nearly identically by all the bodymind disciplines. These
muscles hold *anger*.

Because of the intricate structuring of the human bodymind, nearly all actions are registered in the muscles and
nerve channels of the spine. Conversely, the condition of
the muscles and nerve channels of the spine can be seen to
affect directly the health and well-being of all of the body's
parts and functions. As a result, the structure of the spine
and its functioning potential are often excellent indicators
of the general, as well as the specific, bodymind state of the
individual. In fact, the primary focus of the entire field of

chiropractic medicine is on optimizing the healthy functioning of the spine so that the rest of the body can be vital
as well.[12] Therefore, nearly all forms of bodymind tension
register somewhere along the spine. Conversely, spinal
tension and blockage in turn serve to impair the health of
related organs and limbs. When seen from this perspective,
the healthy flow of energy and grace through the spine is
definitely crucial, for the spine is in a very real sense the
"backbone" of the bodymind.

When feelings are blocked, energy interrupted, expressions thwarted, or action restricted, the energetic charge
often gets deposited somewhere along the spine as well as
in the directly affected bodymind section. As a result, the
spine becomes the "garbage pile" for these unwanted
feelings and unresolved conflicts. By locating themselves
along the spine, the emotions become temporarily
blocked from view, and as they continue to accumulate,
congestion in these muscles increases and the feelings
begin to grow into anger and then rage. If unexpressed,
this rage will translate itself into spite and bitterness,
which will seep into all the expressive aspects of the bodymind in an attempt to release some of the accumulating
tension and conflict. When this happens, the individual is
no longer consciously "in control" of his angry passions.
Instead they have become blocked from consciousness
and from this new place begin themselves to control all
his actions, motions, and expressions.

Several years ago, I had an opportunity to observe a case
in which a huge amount of emotional charge had become
chronically held in someone's shoulders, arms, and upper
back. It was in a five-day encounter therapy group at Esalen, led by Dr. Hector Prestera. On the first night of the
group, all sixteen of us met for several hours to introduce
ourselves and to initiate the encounter process. I was immediately struck by a woman in the group whose name was

Claire. She was so beautiful and sexually attractive that all the men were drawn to her right from the start. As the first days of the workshop passed, each of us hoped that she would be attracted to us.

On the fourth day, a surprise to us all, we discovered that Claire was not at all a swinging single and had, in fact, come to the group with the man with whom she had been living for several years. His name was Robbie. During the first few days of the workshop, neither of them had presented any evidence that they were in any way related to each other outside of Esalen. In that afternoon's session, Robbie walked over to Claire and told her, in front of the whole group, that he was upset that they were not making love. "Big deal," I said to myself. "We all would like to make love with her." Then, as he continued talking, the information came out that, although living together, they had not made love for over three years. That was heavy. Apparently, Claire felt that sex was dirty, and she refused to engage in any sexual activities. It seemed crazy for this unusually attractive woman with her provocative looks and revealing clothing to be averse to sex.

There sat Robbie, quietly explaining to her that he loved her and that he wanted to stroke and embrace her as expressions of his love. His words were calm and rational, yet something else altogether was happening in his body. The group leader spotted it after a few minutes and called Robbie's attention to his shoulders and hands. While he had maintained a peaceful attitude, Robbie's shoulders had drawn back tightly, and as he spoke he continually wrenched and squeezed his clasped hands. Within this calm body lived a raging Godzilla.

The group leader encouraged Robbie to pay attention to the feelings that lived in his shoulders, arms, and back. A large pillow was placed before him and he was instructed to hold the pillow, imagining that it was Claire, and to stroke it/her in any way he would like. Robbie thought this was stupid and wanted to continue debating with Claire as to the rightness or wrongness of sex, but a determined Hector Prestera eventually focused him on the pillow. At first he was self-conscious about his actions and continued to talk to the large pillow as he had previously been talking to Claire . . . quietly. When encouraged to express his feelings with his arms and hands on the pillow, he began to slowly stroke the material and caress its form. The group leader then asked him to stop talking and to express all of his feelings toward Claire nonverbally to the pillow.

The roomful of people was silent and still as everyone curiously observed this man. As we watched, a phenomenal metamorphosis occurred. In all my years of groups and therapy I have never observed such a dramatic and frightening change in any human being. Slowly, as he stroked, his shoulders began to raise and tremble, his arms grew taut, and his hands seemed to swell with tension. This quiet man was gradually transforming himself into a violent constellation of unexpressed rage and violence. As his strokings became tearings and his face grew gnarled, he suddenly began to scream. With the onset of the screaming, he ripped the pillow to pieces and charged after Claire with a look that was murderous. All the men in the group jumped up and grabbed him, attempting to hold him down. For nearly twenty minutes he fought all eight of us in twos, threes, and sixes.

His violence was nearly inexhaustible as he continued to beat all of us with what seemed like mountains of force. Finally, his screaming and rage began to quiet down, and he fell to the floor amidst a pile of exhausted fellow workshop members. His face and arms had grown soft, his breathing steady and full, and his screams of rage had become cries of sadness. Alone, with the group leader close at hand, he proceeded to cry and cry. Some of the other group members cried with him, each of us feeling the pains and frustrations that, in our own private ways, we hold deep within ourselves.

After nearly an hour of what seemed like a purging ritual, Robbie sat up "new." His face was young and light, his shoulders were relaxed and considerably lower than we had ever seen them, and his manner was firm yet soft. He looked at all of us and began to laugh, a laugh that related years of unexpressed anger, sadness, and humor, a laugh that let us know that he had finally released some of what he had been carrying around inside for years.

That session was one of the most frightening yet beautiful experiences I have ever been a part of. It was the sort of release that probably never could have happened except for the unusual set of circumstances that Esalen presents in its encounter workshops. I felt that Hector Prestera handled the session as creatively as a tribal shaman tending to the exorcism of one of his clan. For Robbie, the opportunity to experience and release his feelings offered a chance to get clear with himself about what was really going on inside regarding his own passions as well as his relationship to Claire. The rest of us in the workshop were given an opportunity to see and feel the power of the energy that gets stored in the arms, shoulders, and back, and to get a sense of the way this blocked energy structures our bodies and our minds.

I am not suggesting that this show of emotions carried Robbie off to the promised land or even that it made his life with Claire any more satisfying. Judging from the transformation he experienced during that session and a conversation he and I had later in the week, I felt that the emotional catharsis he experienced had allowed him to release piles of held energy and feelings that had become twisted and jammed within his bodymind. Also, it allowed him to get a clearer and more realistic perspective on himself and his ability to sustain a nourishing, healthy relationship with Claire. His work had just begun, yet he seemed pleased that he was at least beginning with a lighter heart and a lighter hand. The chance for Robbie to release feelings honestly and to come to his senses brought about very much improved self-awareness.

In my own bodymind, the place where I hold a large amount of tension is in the muscles of my upper back. I have come to be aware that this tension relates to the way I hold on to my feelings and relationships with my shoulders and arms. By assuming a continuous posture of psychosomatic vigilance, I create a chronic state of tension in my back. I have learned that when I relax my hold on things and allow the world to flow, the muscles of my back are relieved of some of the stress and I feel considerably more relaxed and comfortable. It's as though I feel that I am carrying the weight of the entire world on my shoulders and that I must hold the ball or else it will (I will) fall apart. By learning to be more trusting and appreciative of others, I am beginning to let go of some of my control. As I do, I am discovering that my back has gotten a bit softer, my arms more gentle, my feelings more balanced, and my heart more available.[13]

CHAPTER

NECK, THROAT, AND JAW

THE NEXT THREE CHAPTERS will present analyses of the bodymind segments that correspond to the fifth, sixth, and seventh chakras. These analyses will differ from those of the first four chakras in that for each chakra region there will be two discussions. First, I will describe some of the psychoemotional functions and potentials of the respective sections of the neck, throat, jaw, face, and skull. Second, I will discuss some of my feelings and experiences in relation to personal growth and self-development, since these three so-called spiritual[1] chakras correspond to the highly developed capacities for thought, language, self-reflection, and self-actualization that separate man from all other creatures. As a result, my examination of these bodymind regions will delve beneath the surface of the skull, inward to an exploration of the unfolding human mind.

By exploring the inner as well as the outer manifestations of these final three chakras, we begin to get a clearer picture of the remarkable evolutionary journey that is implied in the human bodymind.

The bodymind region that corresponds to the fifth Kundalini chakra, "Vishuddha," includes the neck, throat, and jaw. The chakra itself is situated over the throat and connects with the spine at the third cervical vertebra. This bodymind region is primarily concerned with vocal expression and communication. But, in addition, the inner aspects of this chakra center are related to the self-reflective development of an aware self-image, and the throat is said to be the doorway that announces the beginning of an emotional and spiritual ascent into one's inner self. It is here at the throat that you begin to get a clearer, more conscious sense of your relationship both to other people and to yourself. By coming to a more intimate level of communication and expression with yourself, you begin to distinguish your own limits and self-limits, thereby improving your sense of self-identification.[2] This chakra region is therefore concerned with both interpersonal communication and self-identification. Correspondingly, tension in this region might reflect either communication difficulties or conflict in regard to one's self-image. The dual qualities and responsibilities of this region make it doubly interesting as well as doubly difficult to fully diagnose and understand.

THE NECK

Take a few moments to experience your neck. Get a sense of how it feels, what it is shaped like, and what functions it serves with respect to your entire bodymind. Now slowly rotate your neck in order to loosen it up a bit. Go over to a mirror and look at the structure of your neck. See if your neck leans your head off to one side, or if your neck is bent forward. As you rotate your neck in front of the mirror, pay attention to what muscles in your chest, shoulders, and face also stretch with your neck movements. Last, try to imagine what emotional qualities and experiences might correspond to your neck.

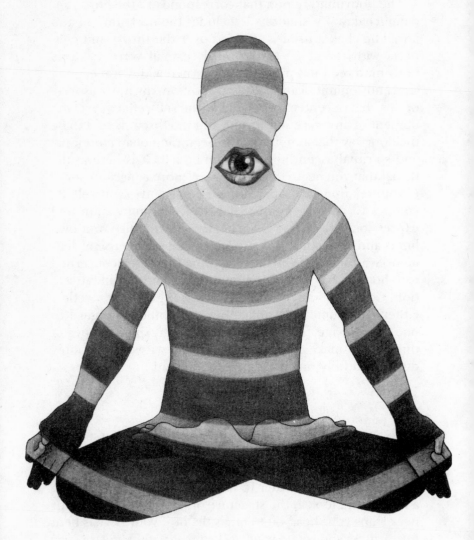

8-1. Fifth Chakra: Throat or Laryngeal Chakra

I can always tell when I am overtired or tense, for my neck will invariably begin to grow stiff and sore. My back and shoulders start to ache a bit, my head begins to droop, and sometimes I can even feel a headache coming on. I notice that my neck is not very discriminating about the type of emotional tension or conflict it responds to. Rather, it seems to be a kind of overall stress barometer, indicating the general degree to which I am either relaxed or tense.

The neck is a fascinating part of the human bodymind for several reasons. First, as emotions flow upward from the belly and chest, they enter the neck, where they are further translated from feelings into thoughts and words. The neck is another processing point along the path of emotional flow through the bodymind. In a way, the neck and throat can be compared to vibrating musical reeds through which life energy and raw emotion pass and are transformed into sounds and concepts. Whereas the chest serves to expand and amplify these emotional flows, it is the neck's function to sort and refine them, dispatching them to their appropriate destinations in the throat and face.

In addition, the neck serves as the major channel through which the brain communicates with the rest of the bodymind. Like a telephone switchboard, the neck provides the energetic linkups between the incoming and outgoing calls.

Because of its structure and position, the neck must continually mediate between feelings and thoughts, impulses and reactions. When the number of calls and communications is more than the emotional and neuromuscular circuits can handle, the lines tend to overload and the bodymind registers a signal, which is immediately felt as tension. When there is a great deal of confusion and conflict in our necks, we feel this blockage as soreness and pain. Tension in the neck can usually be related to a situation in which an individual has taken on more responsibilities than he is able to handle comfortably and gracefully. This informational/ experiential overload registers loud and clear as a "pain in the neck." When such misuse of the neck is continual, the tension becomes a chronic bodymind attitude, at which point the once-flexible neck can become stiff and rigid, thereby limiting its outward motion as well as the flow of impulses and feelings that pass through it.

Because the neck's primary psychosomatic function is that of "mediator," tension in it will often be accompanied by conflict and tension in at least one other important bodymind region. As a result, it is nearly impossible to diagnose the specific nature of the overload simply by visually diagnosing the degree of tension held in the neck. In order to get a clearer understanding of the source of the "overresponsibility" or "inability to cope," the rest of the bodymind must be included in the viewed Gestalt.

For example, I worked with a man several months ago who came to me complaining that he felt completely dissociated from his feelings. Because of this, he was having a great deal of difficulty making decisions about his work and social relationships. We chatted for a while and then I asked him to lie down on his back. After he had done some simple deep breathing and relaxation inductions, I asked him to tell me where he felt the most tension in his body. He immediately responded that his neck was so tight that he felt as though he was wearing an iron collar. This collar was so rigid and tense that he was not able to feel anything in it except continuous pain.

I asked him to breathe slowly and to try to relax and allow an image to come into his mind about the nature of his tight neck. He closed his eyes and became very silent for a few minutes. Then, with a quick laugh, his eyes flashed open, and he told me that he had envisioned his neck as a rope and that his head and torso were having a tug of war with this rope. Apparently, his thoughts and his feelings had chosen up teams that were competing for his attention. This competition was taking place throughout his body-mind with the primary focus in his neck. In his visualization, both teams—thoughts and feelings—were pulling hard on the rope, trying to force the other team across the middle line into the deep pit that separated them.

I told him to assume the personality of each team alternately and then express to me what these teams were fighting for. He immediately became the "thought" team and began talking with a kind of semicontrolled, restrained voice. His breathing was shallow and his body remained quite still. From this perspective he explained how he needed to regain control over his entire self and that the way to assume this control was by blocking off his feelings and placing his thoughts and rational self in charge. Feelings, he said, were a hindrance to his effective functioning because of their unpredictability and manipulative nature. Reason, on the other hand, could be predicted and controlled, allowing more certainty of movement and sureness of position. He was a bright young man and had learned to use his mind extremely well. He felt quite certain that if he could only "beat" his feelings, his life would return to order and the raging thought/feeling conflict in his body-mind would subside.

Then I asked him to mentally become the other team and to share with me what was going on there. Closing his eyes and going inside again, he changed his attitude. His breathing increased, his hands began to move slightly, and his entire body seemed more animated than it had been for the previous few minutes. "I am my feelings," he said. "I am raw, powerful, fiery energy. I have the ability to feel pain, and I am also able to experience pure pleasure." From this perspective, he explained that, while his feelings were somewhat more uncontrolled and stirred up than his thoughts, they were a powerful lot, nevertheless, and would, if allowed to flow uninterrupted, surely bring him feelings of happiness and inner peace. His feelings were upset, however, at having been continually controlled and twisted by his thoughts, and now they were trying to pull his thoughts into the pit, thereby "beating" them and removing the conflict.

The pit that existed between the two teams was described as being "deep, dark, and something entirely horrible." "In a way," he said, "falling into this pit would be like losing control of myself." Each team was trying to force the other into the pit to gain greater control over his bodymind.

I then asked him to imagine what it felt like to be the rope, or his neck, and to share those feelings with me. As he thought about this, his breathing slowed down and he grew sad. When he spoke again, his voice was slow and full. "I wish that my head and body could be on better terms," he said. "I am tired of having them continually fight with each other and I am tired of having to mediate between all their conflicts." As the rope/neck, he reported that what he would like most would be for both teams to take a break from their continual, stressful struggle and to sit down and communicate with each other about not only what they wanted from each other but also what they could do for each other in order to successfully merge teams.

The realization that his neck was suffering all the battle scars from the conflicts raging between his thoughts and feelings saddened him, for it put him in touch with how this battle could never be resolved by a tug-of-war and how one team could never exist without the other. In fact, he really didn't want just one team around without the other to balance it. What he needed to do was to discover ways that he could encourage his thoughts to be a bit more relaxed and respectful of his feelings and his feelings to have some consideration for the needs of his rational mind.

It was clear to both of us that the best way to achieve a higher degree of harmony and cooperation between these two conflicting aspects of himself was to allow each team a chance to get to know the other a little better and to learn to appreciate what the other had to offer it. From the visualization he proceeded to a dialogue between his thoughts and feelings, a dialogue that was no longer a tug-of-war but rather a kind of peacemaking discussion. After quite a bit of bargaining and hassling, the two teams finally came to some mutually agreeable terms. At that point I asked him what his neck felt like. He smilingly reported that, for the first time in months, much of the active tension in his neck was gone, and he felt as though he had been relieved of a great burden.

This short experience seems to be a good example of the role that the neck frequently plays in the development of the bodymind. By acting as the mediator between opposing forces, it tends to accumulate much of the stress of the conflict and can become annoyingly painful and tense. If some aspects of the conflict can be relieved, the neck becomes more able to relax and can then allow the healthy flow of energy upward and downward through the bodymind.

Neck Positions

Rising above the shoulders and torso, the neck also serves as a kind of pedestal upon which the head rests. The shape and positioning of this pedestal, being affected by the types of emotions that animate the related muscles, is frequently indicative of the chronic attitude with which an individual "faces" the world.

For example, put your head out forward so that it extends in front of your body. Now walk around a bit holding your head in this posture. See how you feel when you hold yourself this way.

A head that is chronically held forward usually reflects an individual who encounters the world first with his head, with his rational self, and then later with his body, with his feeling self. The head serves as a kind of psychosomatic search party, racing ahead of the body to survey the landscape and evaluate the psychological conditions before it allows the rest of the wagon train to proceed.

I have also noticed that people tend to lean their heads to one side in conjunction with a particular attitude they are experiencing and projecting. To see what your neck leaning tells you about yourself, tilt your head to one side and try to go inside and see what you feel like when you do this. Then go to a mirror and see what you look like when you do this. Next, lean your head to the other side and once again observe the effect from within and without. These positions might feel and look the same to you, but it is more likely that you will discover that each angle held within it a kind of emotional posturing. When my head is tilted to the right, for example, I find myself feeling arrogant and defiant, as if I have a chip on my shoulder. When I lean to the left, I feel I am projecting a cute and playful attitude. In either case, I don't feel that I am being "straight" but rather that the angling allows me to partly costume my real feelings.

Alexander Lowen points out that "the bearing of the head is in direct relation to the quality and strength of the ego."[3] For example, if the neck and head are bent over forward, "the impression is that the head is too great a burden for the body so it is allowed to droop. This represents the patient's attitude toward reality."[4] This person will have a great deal of difficulty facing up to the demands and needs of everyday living. His head is chronically drooping as a statement of partial defeat and emotional exhaustion.

Similarly, long, graceful necks reflect long, proud attitudes, and stout, bull necks indicate a tight, aggressive approach to life's demands.

As I have said, the neck is responsible for the energetic flow of so many varied feelings and expressions that it is very difficult to read and map it without also referring to other parts of the bodymind. Further, because of its role as emotional mediator, the neck tends to assume the personality of the forces that are at play within it, rather than any one particular quality or type of expression. Therefore, it is hard for me to offer simple diagnostic descriptions for this region. The best way, therefore, to discover what your neck is telling you is to ask it.[5]

THE ORAL SEGMENT:
THROAT, CHIN, AND JAW

The other segment within the domain of the fifth chakra is the so-called oral segment, which includes the structures and functions of the throat, chin, and jaw.

What sort of emotional memories and activities correspond to tension and movement in the oral segment of the face? Since this is the bodymind region that is responsible for a wide variety of expressive actions, such as talking, crying, laughing, biting, smiling, frowning, smelling, eating, spitting, screaming, and swallowing, health and vitality in this region can be seen to correspond to the uninterrupted flow of such actions and emotions. On the other hand, when these actions are restricted from full animation, blockage and tension may result.

According to William Schutz:

> The throat muscles generally hold on to fears of expression. . . . Breathing is held by a tight throat. The child who wanted to yell at his parents but wasn't allowed to held it in his throat so that his voice is strained or too soft. Throat illnesses come easily, coughing is common, and sometimes laughter is stopped prematurely because the tight throat and shallow breathing prevent a true belly laugh; all the laugh must be from the throat upward and attempts to laugh more heartily result in coughing. . . . Fear of inclusion is often accompanied by a tight throat and a soft, unintelligible voice. . . . This is consistent with the throat chakra being the center of communication.
>
> The bottom of the jaw is often the place where tears are held from prematurely stopped crying. . . . The jaw muscle

itself (masseter) often holds much anger due to biting inhi-
bitions when young. . . . Dental problems caused by exces-
sive grinding (bruxion) are often traceable to repressed
anger. The position of the lower jaw is determined largely
by the tightness of the masseter. This means that if a small
child were unable to speak up to his parents, he would tend
to hold back on his jaw muscle, thus pulling his lower jaw
back. This results in an overbite (buck teeth) and sometimes
a lisp, since the upper and lower teeth must be almost
together to make a proper "s" sound.[6]

I have been continually amazed at the quantity of emotional experience that gets locked in the jaw, throat, and
mouth. It's hard to believe that such a small bodymind
region contains so many large expressions, feelings, and
memories.

Several years ago, I was co-leading a workshop at Esalen
with Will Schutz. The workshop was entitled "Bodymind"
and was a combination of encounter and Feldenkrais work.
During one of the encounter sessions, a woman in the
group expressed an interest in working on some tension
that she regularly felt in her throat and jaw. She was an
unusually heavy woman, with an underactive thyroid, due,
I believe, to all the repressed crying and screaming that she
held in her throat; she was a chain smoker; and she seemed
to have difficulty expressing her feelings. At the time that
she chose to try to work on her condition, we were all nude
and were into our fourth day of encountering.

She and I moved into the center of the room, and she
began trying to explain to me why she smoked so much and
why she felt so much tension in her jaw. There was no need
for her to verbalize, for the tension was obvious to me in
her receding jaw and raspy voice. I decided to use a bioenergetic exercise to release the holding in her throat. Placing
the end of a towel in her mouth, I asked her to bite down
hard on it, while I held the other end of the towel and
pulled on it against her resistance. This particular tech-

nique increases the muscle tension in the throat and jaw, thereby exaggerating the feelings, thus making therapeutic work easier. Well, I pulled and pulled, and she tugged and tugged—for nearly ten minutes.

Finally, she began to gag and cough. As she did so, her throat and mouth began to vibrate and quiver. I encouraged her to express whatever emotions she felt and to try not to block her feelings. After a few moments her wailings turned into words, and we all listened as she screamed violently at her father whom she hadn't seen for several years. For nearly thirty minutes she yelled at him and cursed him for all the mean and insensitive ways he had treated her throughout her life. It seemed as though she had always wanted to tell him off and yell at him in the way he had apparently always yelled at her. Yet she was afraid of what the consequences might be if she ever let him have some of her "lip."

It was wonderful to watch the changes that occurred throughout her entire bodymind as she unloaded the emotional garbage that had been stuck in her throat for so long. After her screaming and wailing ceased, she cried a bit in rediscovery of herself.

It's hard to tell what long-range effects that session may have had on her life, but my guess is that this oral release must have lightened her load a bit as she learned how to express her negative emotions. The quality and texture of her voice changed during the workshop, and I noticed she didn't smoke for the rest of the week. During the last few days of the workshop, her emotional state was light and airy, and she seemed considerably more relaxed and in touch with herself than she had been before this catharsis.

Violence and anger are not the only emotions that are held in the jaw. In fact, nearly any emotion that is expressed through either the mouth or face can become fixed in the armor of the throat and jaw.[11] In another Esalen workshop, I had an opportunity to observe a fascinating example of another type of emotional holding that frequently locates itself in the oral segment of the bodymind.

The workshop was called "Freeing the Body" and was led by Dr. Hector Prestera. In it there was a young, attractive woman named Anna, who was rather quiet and withdrawn. Several times during the workshop she became involved in emotional encounters, but each time she seemed to be partially removed from the feelings of the moment. When she cried, she only whimpered, and when she spoke, it was always in a reserved and restrained fashion. All her expressions were somewhat monotonous, and she seemed to be holding all her verbalizations and emotions down deep inside her. For days, Hector encouraged her to express her feelings in order to get down to whatever it was that was troubling her, but each time she only went so far and then stopped herself. Finally, on the last night of the workshop she began talking about her family, and Hector immediately spotted her jaw freezing up.

He quickly moved over to her and began Rolfing her jaw.[7] As he worked on her jaw, her chest began to swell, and before long her breathing was heavy and emotion-laden. She began to cry and cry. This time she was really crying, not at all like the whimpers that we had heard before. I don't know how he knew what was happening, but in a flash Hector had understood the nature of her tears and had constructed a psychodrama[8] with the help of the other members of the group.

An improvised stage was immediately set with dim lights, and one of the group members lay still in the middle of the room as though he were dead. Anna looked at the situation and slowly moved over to the "dead" person and began talking to him. For a long time, she expressed her love and caring for this dead person, whom she called Jimmy, and told him things she had apparently wanted to tell him for years. She wept as she stroked the dead boy's face and cried violently with long-held love for him. As she continued to talk to Jimmy, we learned that this was her little brother, who had been killed in a car accident seven years before when he was just ten years old. Anna had held herself partly responsible for his death, for he had been struck down on an afternoon when she was supposed to be watching out for him.

It was clear that she had held mountains of guilt for her little brother's death for all those years. To compound the tension, she had not been permitted to cry or to speak to the dead child at his funeral. Her parents kept her away from the coffin, telling her that such emotions and actions would embarrass them. So for all those years, her chest, throat, and jaw had been filled up with unexpressed feelings and expressions. Hector tenderly guided her through the drama, allowing her to say and do all the things to her little brother that she had not been able to do during the real funeral ceremony. Finally, Anna let go of the last of her held feelings and said goodbye to Jimmy. Only then did she seem to be ready to acknowledge his passing—and at the same moment acknowledge the energy of her own life.

That evening was a very touching and somber one for each of us, for it seemed that we all had feelings and loves that we had not expressed to people we cared about, both alive and dead. We all cried and in our own ways joined Anna in saying goodbye to her brother, and in doing so allowed ourselves to appreciate the freshness of "now" and the beauty of being alive and open enough to share our lives with other people.

During the five years since this experience I have been a part of a great many encounter and psychodrama situations where people expressed some of the feelings that they had not been able to express at the passing of loved ones. These thoughts and emotions frequently become blocked in the jaw and throat, thereby interrupting the natural flow of energy through this region and restricting all expression. If these emotions ever become "uncorked," so to

speak, there is often a freeing up of many of the emotions
and experiences that have become trapped behind the tension of the initial trauma.

The variety of ways in which the oral segment of the face
can position itself are countless, and the variety of emotions and experiences that structure these bodily attitudes
are also countless. In general, however, tension in the jaw
reflects some degree of blockage of the expression of either
emotions or verbal communications. The three most common forms of chronic tension in this region are manifested
in a receding jaw, a protruding jaw, or a clenched jaw
(which might exist in combination with one of the other
two).

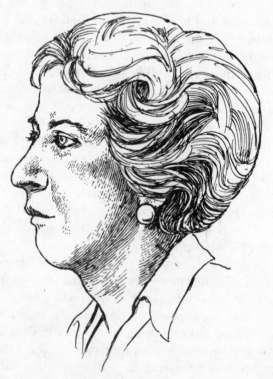

8-2. *Receding Jaw*

Receding Jaw

A receding jaw usually reflects withheld sadness or anger, or an urge to cry or scream. This blockage may hamper an individual's ability to express any of his emotions and beliefs orally, whether they relate to the emotion that caused the freeze in the body's growth or not. This person might tend to have a great deal of difficulty speaking up in groups, defending himself, and voicing his opinion.

Protruding Jaw

A forward protrusion of the jaw, on the other hand, reflects a defiant character attitude. When the jaw is slightly forward it indicates that the person has an extremely "determined" way of being in the world. It is almost as though he were trying to pull himself forward with the thrust of his jaw. As the position of the jaw moves farther forward, the determined attitude becomes increasingly one of defiance and arrogance.

Clenched Jaw

I believe that a clenched jaw is an indication of over-self-control. When I catch myself clenching my jaw (I often do it unconsciously), it is usually at a time when there is a great deal that I want to say or express but I am holding on to it. It is almost as if I think that by clenching my jaw I can swallow or dissolve the emotion or information that has made its way to my mouth.

As is true of the neck, the oral segment is psychosomatically related to a large variety of feelings, and it is also a difficult region of the bodymind to read accurately or quickly from the outside. When I diagnose jaw blockage, I also pay attention to the person's breathing, chest struc-

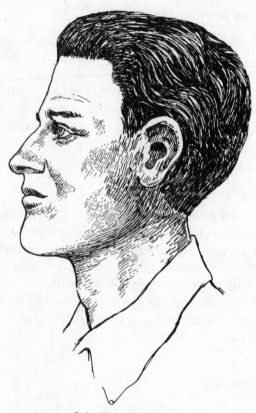

8-3. *Protruding Jaw*

ture, pelvic positioning, and speech pattern in order to get a picture of the overall personality and the sorts of feelings that he might be comfortable expressing or not expressing. I have found that since the jaw is responsible for expressing a great many feelings that actually originate in other parts of the bodymind, tension in the jaw is usually developed in conjunction with some other related bodymind part.

For example, I am working at present with a thirty-year-old man who is a chronic stutterer. He came to me with the hope of relieving the tension that he continually felt in his throat and jaw. He had been stuttering severely for twenty-five years. My initial response was to work on his jaw, mouth, and throat, for there was obvious tension and blockage in this region. After several weeks of neck massage and Reichian breathing work, I discovered something fascinating about his stuttering. He didn't actually stutter from his throat and jaw; rather, the stuttering originated in his diaphragm and belly. This might be difficult to imagine, but what happened when he stuttered was that, before the words actually got to his face, his diaphragm went into a quick spasm which interrupted the natural flow of air and energy upward to his mouth. The diaphragmatic interruption was then translated into the words that flowed interruptedly through his jaw. The more we worked together, the more I saw that most of the tension in his jaw resulted from the simple fact that he had been trying to squeeze broken words out of his throat for years with no success. Normal speech was impossible. By practicing deep breathing and by releasing, through yoga and bioenergetic exercises, some of the rage that apparently lived in his diaphragm, we have together discovered that he can create a more balanced flow of energy through his body, thereby considerably diminishing the stuttering effect when he speaks.[9]

I have since come to a fuller appreciation of the jaw, not as an emotion originator but as an emotion translator and communicator. To perceive the initial source of jaw tension, therefore, you must explore the entire bodymind dynamic.[10]

SELF-IDENTIFICATION

Throughout this book, I have repeatedly pointed out the relationships between specific body parts and the emotional memories and feelings that seem to live within these parts. When we begin to explore the topography of the mind, however, the easy-to-observe muscles, bones, and organs become replaced by not-so-easy-to-observe thoughts, images, and concepts, which to a large extent are the muscles and bones that hold the skeletons of our psyches together. As a result, my discussions of these inner terrains will focus on the way we shape and form our minds and beliefs.

The fifth Kundalini chakra, "Vishuddha," in addition to being responsible for vocal expression and interpersonal communication, corresponds to the uniquely human powers of self-reflection and self-identification. It is here that we begin to develop an honest inner voice with which we converse inwardly with ourselves. This region is more concerned with inward communicating, inward looking, inward feeling, inward sensing, inward exploring, and inward knowing than were the previously discussed regions, whose focus was to a large extent on outward contact and interpersonal relationships. At the level of the fifth chakra, we begin to take greater advantage of the fact that as humans we possess the ability to reflect on ourselves, to evaluate our condition, and to initiate action to alter our bodyminds and lives if we so decide. It seems quite fitting that the drives and passions of the first four chakras—grounding and survival needs; sexual drives and primary interpersonal relationships; raw emotion, power, and social identification; compassion, love, and self-expression—should be explored and developed before the bodymind emphasis begins to shift from matters of survival and interpersonal exchange to those of self-reflection and conscious self-identification. In addition, it also seems appropriate that self-reflection and self-identification should precede the qualities of the sixth and seventh chakra regions, which focus on expanded mental powers, heightened self-awareness, and self-realization.

The fifth chakra is considered the first "spiritual" chakra, for it marks the beginning of an individual's deeper understanding of his own relationship to himself. At this point in the evolution of human be-ing, the power and passion of the lower levels are turned inward on oneself, where they supply the energy and drive for self-understanding and spiritual awakening.

Who are you? What do you know about yourself? Are you healthy? What do you feel? How do you feel? What are your strengths? your weaknesses? Are you satisfied with who you are? What do you believe? Are you happy? Does your self-image please you? Are there ways that you could know more about yourself? Are you being suffocated by your habits? Are you what you want to be, or are you what others want you to be? Can you discover ways to further explore your human potential?

In my own life, I have been struggling with these questions in an attempt to understand more fully who and what I am, so that I can allow myself to lead the fullest, most vital life possible. I believe that I have the best chance for actualizing my dreams if I first come to really appreciate my uniqueness, my history, my strengths, my weaknesses, my self.

The first time I ever consciously sat down with myself and tried to look inward was in 1968, when at the age of eighteen, after having successfully completed my freshman year of college as a budding electrical engineer, I had a curious realization. It occurred to me that I had only a very small idea as to *who* or *what* I was. Oh sure, I knew what I looked like, and how I scored on aptitude tests, and that I needed work on my tennis backhand, and that some people liked me, and that I sometimes made my parents proud of me by achieving well in academic, athletic, and social activities, and that I was good at certain things and not so good at other things, and that some women found me attractive and others didn't. I also knew a bit about calculus, sociology, literature, physics, economics, manners, and a variety of rules and requirements for all sorts of games and situations. Yet I didn't know all that much about *me*. Most of what I had come to define as aspects of myself, I had learned *from the outside in* rather than *from the inside out*, so when it came right down to it, almost all I knew about myself was how well I performed and how I appeared to other people.

All this learning from the outside in was focused on my ability to master bits of information and specific skills. When I studied a subject, I studied it in order to get a good grade; when I exercised my body, I did so in order to make it either run faster or perform better. When I became old enough to develop my own personality, I chose one that I thought people would like and be attracted to. I worked very hard at training myself to look and act like a wonderful person, and at the age of eighteen I already could look back upon a fruitful life of loving friendships, academic accomplishment, and athletic achievement. I suppose I was a version of the all-American boy.

Yet it was painfully clear to me that I had been living my life entirely in response to what others wanted from and for me, and that I was almost completely detached from my own interests, passions, and dreams. As a result, there was a hollowness to my feelings. My happiness seemed to be more related to success and achievement than it was to my own inner feelings of satisfaction and self-worth. My actions were motivated by the responses I anticipated, and in this regard my feelings were as much a part of my outer costume as was my clothing. I realized that, powerful and charismatic as I seemed to be on the outside, on the inside I was a good deal less sure of myself. This condition was due to the schism that existed within me, between what I was doing and how I was doing it, between my outer shell and my inner core, between what I had learned about myself through outer actions and what I had learned about myself through inner explorations. It was not that I was avoiding my own initiatives but rather that I had never given myself time to discover what they were.

When it suddenly struck me at the age of eighteen that I was somewhat of a stranger to myself, and that the inner parts of me were only marginally related to the outer parts of me, my immediate reaction was panic. My fear was partly due to the fact that I could no longer live my life as a puppet on my own strings, and partly due to the realization that I didn't really know how to live my life any other way.

For several years I blundered, going frantically from one experience to another, one mood to another, one personality to another, trying on personalities as I used to try on sport jackets, hoping that I would somehow find one that fitted. These years were hard and painful ones for me; I found myself without a sense of self, starkly alone for the first time in my life, and embarrassingly confused about what I was supposed to be doing with my life. No matter what I tried, all I seemed to discover was more unhappiness and confusion. During that time, my physical health was terrible and I seemed to be as tormented in my body as I was in my mind. My body grew rigid and fragile, I was continually suffering from sore throats and viruses, I frequently felt faint and afraid for no apparent reason. It was as though I had removed the bodymind mask that I had been wearing all my life without having another one to replace it with, leaving myself weak and vulnerable.

I never really "found" myself by frantically trying to assume a different personality, but those years of existential conflict and confusion did allow me to begin to see the way I had come to form myself and so presented a variety of clues about how I might begin to redevelop myself into a more self-aware, more conscious being. One of the things I had realized was that my self-image was almost entirely made up of information I had received from sources other than myself, such as parents, friends, teachers, books, and the media. It became clear to me that if I was going to revise my self-image, I would have to begin exploring myself and my world through my own senses and perceptions.

It was at this time that I became involved with the various

techniques and processes of the embryonic human-potential movement. I was immediately fascinated by the emphasis on self-responsibility, experiential learning, and self-discovery that underlies most of these methods and practices. It was my hope that by exploring and examining the various aspects of my bodymind with activities such as encounter groups, yoga, meditation, and Rolfing, I would begin to realize who and what I *really* was. I was in desperate need of some education from the inside out to balance all that I had received from the outside in.

I feel that my curiosities and hopes have been well satisfied, for when I began to identify and isolate the forces, experiences, habits, and preferences that merged to form my unique bodymind, I not only became more aware of my limits and potentials but I also discovered that with the appropriate sensitivity and tools, I could begin to recreate myself in a more healthy, more vital, more conscious fashion.

By learning to maintain a healthy balance between all that I had been taught and programmed to believe about myself, on the one hand, and all that I was beginning to discover about myself through my own inner journeys and bodymind explorations on the other, I found that a "new" and considerably more self-aware "me" was beginning to emerge. Apparently, by simultaneously letting go of some of my social programming while at the same time discovering my true feelings, passions, and potentials through self-dialogue, experiential exercises, and introspective activities, I had begun to allow myself to come alive . . . perhaps for the first time.

I have since become fascinated with the ways in which people develop self-images that are either unattached to their real selves, dishonest, or destructively limiting. Correspondingly, I am especially interested in techniques and methods that bring people into more direct and honest contact with themselves.

While there are thousands of ways a person might constructively educate and nourish his overall self-image, I would like to take a few moments to discuss one system that works primarily with the body. This is the method for bodymind awareness that has been developed by Moshe Feldenkrais, an Israeli physicist with a wide range of experience in both physical and mental approaches to self-understanding. Since Feldenkrais's approach to self-awareness offers a valuable perspective on the ways in which self-image relates to bodymind development, and since it corresponds closely to the nature and focus of the fifth chakra, I have decided to incorporate some of his perspectives into my discussion of this bodymind region.

Feldenkrais and Self-Image

Feldenkrais's perspective is simple yet profound. He believes that the bodymind, being continually influenced by hereditary, cultural, and personal factors, develops a constellation of physical, emotional, and intellectual habit patterns that collectively define the self-image of the individual. He points out that while these habit patterns surely serve their respective functions, they can also be limiting and restrictive and may ultimately keep an individual from making fuller use of himself.[11]

For example, fold your hands together. Experience how they feel. Then, unfold them and refold them the other way. How do they feel now? Relax your arms and then fold them across your chest and experience the way this feels. Then, unfold them and refold them, reversing the position of your arms. How does this feel?

Chances are that, in both cases, one way was more usual, more comfortable, more "you" than the other way, which, while equally simple and legitimate, felt awkward and alien. Some of you might not have been able to place your hands or arms in any but your accustomed positions.

This is a simple example, on the somatic level, of Feldenkrais's perspective. He suggests that similar preferences, biases, and habits also exist on the emotional and intellectual levels. While Feldenkrais is the first to admit that habits and regular bodymind patterns are necessary elements of day-to-day living, he reminds us that the exploration and development of our unused potential often lies past the borders of these self-restrictive limits and beliefs.

In response to the physical, emotional, intellectual, and experiential limits imposed on the bodymind, and therefore on all aspects of the individual's self-image, Feldenkrais has devised thousands of movement exercises and activities that are designed to encourage people to become more aware of themselves and their potential.[12] The exercises are so unusual in their form and practice that they force people to explore and integrate aspects of themselves that have probably been out of their awareness for years. He believes that by working directly with the neuromuscular connections of the bodymind, one can increase one's self-awareness and enhance one's self-image, allowing a greatly enhanced sense of control over oneself.

The various Feldenkrais exercises are designed to allow you to move yourself and experience yourself in unusual and sometimes difficult ways. There is no right or wrong way to do the exercises, for performance in any particular fashion is not the aim. Rather, by doing the exercises and by paying attention to yourself as you do, you begin to send new messages to your nervous system, which, in turn, sends new messages back to your muscles. Feldenkrais suggests that many of the limitations to greater bodymind awareness and flexibility originate in the nervous system and are then projected into the muscles and connective tissue. His exercises therefore place greater emphasis on freeing up the nervous system than on stretching the muscles. By breaking up your usual neuromuscular patterns, you begin to train yourself to think, move, feel, and sense in more expansive ways than you are accustomed to. Feldenkrais's belief is that the bodymind will continually reorganize itself to accommodate new and more useful information. As a result, the more aware you are throughout your entire bodymind, the more able you will be to organize and use yourself efficiently, effectively, and consciously.

Here in condensed form, is an example of a Feldenkrais bodymind exercise:

Stand with your right arm extended straight out in front of you at shoulder level. Look at your right hand and turn your arm, head, and eyes together to the right as far as they will go without strain. Note a point on the wall corresponding to that distance. Now swing back slowly to the front position. Let your arm down and relax. . . . Raise it again to the front position. Move your arm to the right as before, but at the same time, move your head to the left. Move both head and arm as far as you can without strain. Do this five times, returning to the center position between trials. Be aware of the feelings in your neck, shoulders, and waist during these five movements. Put your arm down and relax. . . . Now once again try the original motion of raising your arm, looking at your hand, and moving your arm, head, and eyes to the right as far as they will go without strain. Compare it with the original point on the wall. You will probably observe that you moved considerably farther. Put your arm down and relax. . . . Again put your arm in the front position. Now move your arm to the right and your head and hips (pelvis) to the left, all as far as they will go without strain. Do this five times, returning to the center position between trials. Be very aware of all your body movements. Put your arm down and relax. . . . Again try the original movement, moving your arm to the right as far as you can without strain. Compare the distance your arm now travels with the original distance. It is probable that your arm turns noticeably farther to the right than it did before. Come back to the center, put your arm down and relax.

Now hold your left arm straight out in front, look at your

left hand and turn your head, trunk, and arm to the left as far as you can without strain and note the point on the wall. Come back to the front. Put your arm down. Relax. . . . Put it up again in the front position. Now *only in your imagination,* repeat the first movements made with the right arm three times each. That is, imagine your left arm going left and your head going right, three times. Then imagine your arm going left and and your head and hip going right three times. While you do this, concentrate on the muscle feelings. Try to see three clear movements. After the imagined movement, open your eyes, put your arm down, and relax. . . . Now put your left arm in front as before, look at your hand, and move your arm, trunk, and head to the left and note the difference in the point on the wall. There will probably be almost as large an increment as with the right side, although it was gained without any movement. [Italics in original.][13]

What I especially appreciate about Feldenkrais's method is his unflagging emphasis on self-experience and self-reflection as paths toward greater self-knowledge, and his belief that self-limiting bodymind habits and behaviors keep us from developing large portions of our untapped potentials. The Feldenkrais exercises emphasize no particular goal, no perfect body, no ideal person. Rather this bodymind method seeks only to allow its practitioner as many opportunities as possible to become more intimately aware of himself through creative exercises, visualizations, and unusual movements. By increasing the neuromuscular connections in his bodymind, the Feldenkrais practitioner develops a more expansive self-image and so becomes able to organize himself more efficiently and thereby realize new, more pleasurable possibilities for graceful and free movement of his body.[14]

Now, I am not about to suggest that our self-images are not heavily influenced by hereditary and cultural factors, for they surely are. Each of us is born into a genetic code, a family, a community, a culture, and a time that offer certain definite possibilities and certain definite restrictions. Nevertheless, I believe that no matter what your particular life situation is, there are probably ways, no matter how seemingly minor and menial, in which you can begin to explore the possibility of using yourself more creatively, more healthfully, and with greater self-awareness.

I have discovered in my own bodymind that many of my habits and preferences are not necessarily due to any major commitment or physical deficiency but rather to a lack of involvement in new and stimulating activities. The forces of laziness and the easy way out all too often outweigh the more risky routes of change and development. In our culture of instant everything, it's pretty simple to just slip into a comfortable set of patterns and become trapped and fixed within their structures.

For example, I recently decided to paint several of the rooms in my house. After I began spreading the paint, I noticed that my arm was getting tired, so I tried switching the brush over to my left hand. At first, I was put off by my own awkwardness of movement in this arm, and my immediate response was to take the brush back into my right hand again, no matter how exhausted it was getting. Then I stopped myself and decided that I would try to learn how to paint with my left hand as comfortably as I had always done with my right. It didn't come easy at first, but after a while I found that either arm could be used for the execution of this simple household task. This process of growth involved first discovering my limitation and then allowing myself a chance to transcend it.

This same process of exploring and expanding self-limits was exemplified on the level of personality and personal values several years ago in an incident that took place between my father and me. One summer while I was living in Big Sur, California, and working at Esalen Institute, my parents decided to get on a plane and come out to visit me. My parents are from New Jersey and have lived there all their lives. As a result, they have become accustomed to the styles of behavior, dress, and action that predominate in and around the neighborhoods where they live and work. Naturally, the patterns of their lives have been shaped by the unique cultural factors that characterize a normal life in that region of the country.

Yet, there they were on one sunny summer afternoon, standing on the lawn at Esalen Institute among the long-haired, seminude, hippie-like populace of the Esalen live-in community. It was quite a cultural shock for my father, who with his expensive slacks and white shoes felt entirely out of place among the blue jeans and bare feet. In a way, the initial exposure to another "culture" gave him an idea of the way I always feel when I fly back to New Jersey and try to fit into their home and life style.

My father's first reaction was to call all the people "wackos." He nervously made fun of the way they looked and at what they were doing with themselves, while continuously criticizing them for living their lives in such an "unproductive" fashion. It was clear that his beliefs and habits were crashing up against his own limits, which were being intensely confronted by another set of styles and possibilities.

Yet as the days wore on, giving my parents an opportunity to relax a bit and to communicate with many of the curiously lovely Esalen residents, a change began taking place in my father's belief system. When he realized that these were people like himself who were simply trying to be happy and lead nourishing lives, he suddenly stopped his criticisms and grew quiet for several days as he seemed to be revaluating some of his beliefs. Finally, on the last day of their visit, we were sitting on a beautiful cliff overlooking the majestic Pacific Ocean and my father said to me, "You know, it's easy to get used to a certain set of rules and habits, and when you do, you get a little frightened of people and places that don't fit into your world view. Maybe one way is really not any better than another . . . but maybe each of us needs to find a way of living and being that most nourishingly fits our needs and preferences. I personally couldn't live out here on the side of a mountain, and it would make me very uncomfortable and unhappy to do so, but I can see that the people here would be just as uncomfortable if they tried to live my life and walk in my shoes."

This realization of my father's not only served to strengthen the bonds of respect that exist between us but also helped to illustrate how many of our beliefs and attitudes are simply a result of habit and exposure. We all become most familiar and comfortable with those physical, intellectual, and emotional aspects of ourselves with which we are most frequently in contact and communication.

These types of experiences suggest that our self-images, and our bodyminds and lives, are largely a result of the patterns of behavior and movement that we have developed for ourselves and that we practice regularly.[15] All too often it is exactly these self-propagated limits and habits that rigidify our minds, prohibiting the flow of creative thought, and tighten our bodies, denying its pleasures. By truly realizing the way we do this to ourselves, each of us stands a chance to improve and expand our lives and awaken some of our untapped potential.

The further conclusion I draw is that with the heightened self-knowledge gained through self-experience and self-reflection, we can learn to construct our bodyminds and lives so as to allow the development of increased health, vitality, and consciousness. It is this human quality, the ability to mindfully reflect on one's own existence, and to generate change in that existence, that epitomizes the self-identifying aspects of the fifth Kundalini chakra. For as self-perceivers, we not only breathe air into our lungs, we also have the ability to breathe imagination into our thoughts and consciousness into our lives.

FACE AND HEAD

THE OCULAR SEGMENT of the face, which includes the ears, the eyes, the forehead, and the cheekbone region, corresponds to the sixth Kundalini chakra, "Ajna," which is located on the forehead between the eyebrows and is related to the development of heightened self-awareness. When added to the oral segment, the ocular segment makes up the region of our bodyminds that we call our *face*, and so I would like to build on the information I presented on the jaw in the last chapter as I continue to explore some of the ways in which our faces reflect our inner natures.[1] According to Alexander Lowen:

> [The face] is the part of the body that is openly presented to the world. It is also the first part examined when one looks at another person. . . . The word "face" is also used to refer to a person's image which relates the concept of face to ego, since the ego in one of its functions is concerned with the image a person projects. "To lose face." If one "hides his face," it denotes a sense of shame in which the ego feels humiliated. A person with a strong ego "faces

up" to situations, while a weaker person might "face away." Self-expression involves the face, and the kind of face we put on ourselves tells a great deal about who we are and how we feel. There is the smiling face, the depressed face, the bright face, the sad face, etc. Unfortunately most people are unaware of the expression on their faces and to that extent are out of touch with who they are and how they feel.[2]

As Lowen suggests, your face is the mask that you present to the world, and it therefore reveals quite a bit about your inner feelings. I also think that in addition to shaping our faces as a result of who we actually are and how we are actually feeling, we also shape our faces as a result of who we pretend to be and how we pretend to be feeling. Therefore, when there is conflict between our true nature and our make-believe nature, this conflict will frequently register in the muscles of our faces as tension. For example, think of what you do with your face when you are around people whom you dislike but nevertheless act as though you liked. Chances are, when you are in this situation, your face displays a kind of plastic smile and tense attentiveness, while on the inside you're growling and frowning. If you were to act this conflict out, you'd probably notice that when you hold yourself this way a great deal of tension quickly accumulates in all the muscles of your face and neck.

Several days ago I had to go to the California Department of Motor Vehicles to renew my driver's license and found myself in a situation that clearly exemplifies some of the function of the "face." After I had taken the written test and the eye test, I was asked to go over to the camera so they could take a picture of me for my new license. I had not been expecting to have my picture taken, so I immediately rushed off into the bathroom to make sure that my hair looked just right and my face was in order. I then tried to decide how I wanted to appear in this picture, for it would be identifying me for years to come. Should I show my intellectual face, or my happy face? My sexy face or my serious face? In order to see which face would be most appropriate for my license photograph, I spent about fifteen minutes standing in front of the bathroom mirror slowly trying all of them on to see which one fitted the best. As I was doing this I realized that, in a less conscious way, I do this very same thing hundreds of times each day. That is, as I encounter different people and different situations, I frequently make my face assume a shape that will display the emotional tone that I want to project, whether I am feeling it or not. Now, I am not saying that I do this all the time, for there are surely occasions when my feelings and actions are entirely spontaneous and my facial expressions honestly display my true emotions, but there definitely are other times when my face is more like a mask that I consciously shape in order to pretend to the world that I am feeling what I'm really not.

I find that I control my face in this fashion most frequently when I am trying to cover up some emotion that I have decided not to express. For example, let's say that I am at a party and I go up to an attractive woman and ask her to dance. In response to my somewhat nervous request, she replies that she would rather not dance with me. I immediately feel rejected, embarrassed, and hurt. On the inside, I feel my entire bodymind responding to the jolt of her denial, and if I were to let my face respond freely, my bright smile and open face might suddenly be replaced by a quivering jaw and crying eyes. Yet, determined to stay cool, I smile back at her with a phony grin and hard eyes, attempting to project the impression that I am not bothered.

This is a good example of how, by covering up emotions and presenting a false image to other people, I freeze tension into the muscles of my face. The muscles I am dishonestly controlling are, in fact, registering my internal conflicts as the tension in them builds and becomes locked into the related musculature. As is the case with every other area of my bodymind, if I sustain this conflict long enough, it will become a chronic structuring of my muscles, and I will have developed a bodymind armor that could determine the future health, vitality, and expressiveness of this region.

Armoring in the muscles of the ocular segment can also be the result of a traumatic experience, one so powerful that it locks the muscles into a chronic state of contraction that reflects the power and intensity of the initial encounter. A perfect example of this type of blockage is in *Tommy,* an opera written and performed by the rock group The Who.

In this story, a young man and woman fall in love and get married. Shortly after their wedding, the husband is called off to war, leaving the young wife, who is now pregnant, alone. While he is away, the woman gives birth to a boy whose name is Tommy. When the war ends and the father does not return home, the wife receives information that he has been lost in the line of duty. Assuming him dead, she finds a new lover who cares for her and also fathers the growing boy.

Then one night, as the woman and her lover are asleep in bed, the father returns home. First stopping in his son's room to kiss the boy, he walks in on his unsuspecting wife and her lover. In rage and panic, the lover kills the father with a blow on the head. But while all this is happening, Tommy is standing silently in the doorway, observing everything. When the mother and lover realize that Tommy has seen and heard the whole horrible murder, they scream at him, demanding that he lose his memory of the entire occurrence. In response, the otherwise healthy boy immediately becomes deaf, dumb, and blind. Only much later in life, after a fantastic collection of experiences, does

Tommy finally emerge from his internal hiding place to regain full use of his sensory capacities.

This story is perfectly illustrative of the way in which many of us apparently become traumatized early in our lives by experiencing activities that are so frightening or painful that we respond by shutting off the feelings directly at their source, in many cases at a specific bodymind part or organ. Varying degrees of this type of traumatic blockage are, in fact, quite ordinary, and are treated frequently in bioenergetic, Reichian, and other therapies.[3]

Whether facial tension or armoring is due to present psychoemotional conflicts or past unresolved emotional trauma, the fact remains that it exists and plagues a great many of us. Tension in the ocular segment of the face is usually located in the region that functionally registers the conflict; conflict in regard to hearing is often situated in the region of the ears; in regard to seeing, around the eyes; and so on.

Every part of your face tells stories about your unique life and personal history. In fact, there is a special diagnostic science called physiognomy[4] that aims to evaluate complex social and medical phenomena in the shape, form, and texture of the face. For my purposes in this book, however, I will discuss only three bodymind regions within the ocular segment of the face: the ears, the eyes, and the forehead.

THE EARS

The ears are used primarily for hearing, plain and simple. When you decide that you "don't want to hear it any more," you will probably begin to withdraw your attention from this bodymind region, thereby decreasing awareness of your ears and diminishing your ability to hear. In addition, your difficulty in hearing will probably be accompanied by tension in the various neuromuscular regions that surround your ears, and at this point you will truly turn off your ability to hear what other people have to say to you. While many loss-of-hearing and ear problems surely come from genetic weaknesses and purely physical damage, I have discovered, especially while working with older people, that hearing is as much a psychosocial activity as it is a purely physiological function. People often hear just as much as they wish to hear for just as long as they want to hear it; after that point, they may begin to develop hearing difficulties. When this psychosomatic attitude becomes habitual, permanent hearing loss may be the outcome.

For example, several years ago, at the age of eighty-three, my grandfather died. He was quite a wonderful man, unique in his simplicity and admirable for the respect he showed to all the members of our family. In return, we all loved him dearly, yet no one loved him more than my grandmother. At the time of his death they had been happily married for fifty-nine years. Quite a team they were, fitting together like a hand in a glove. I loved to be around them, for after so many years of being together they functioned smoothly and gracefully as a single unit, each one fitting into the other's grooves, sharing strengths as well as weaknesses, pain as well as joy.

Now, it's important to be aware that my grandparents were not terribly sociable and that, aside from visiting with family members, they spent a great deal of the past twenty years alone except for each other; they seemed to be living each day for one another and experiencing each moment only to share it with the other. When my grandfather died, an interesting thing happened to my grandmother's hearing. Before his death she had been able to hear everything that my grandfather or anyone else said to her. When he died, however, she immediately became nearly deaf.

If she were to be examined by a doctor, he would no doubt say that her hearing loss was due to the fact that she was old and that her ears were giving out on her. Yet I know differently, for from where I sit, when my grandfather died, everything worth listening to left with him. It is almost as if she had made a conscious decision to turn off her ears once she knew she couldn't hear him speak to her again. My grandmother was not a talkative or social woman, and hearing has not been a crucial element in her interpersonal relationships . . . except when there was someone with whom she wanted to talk and share herself. After my grandfather was gone, she apparently decided that she would rather put her attention elsewhere.

I have observed this same phenomenon scores of times while working with older people in nursing homes and rest homes. Many of the people who live in these residences could be described as both hard of hearing and senile, and the interpersonal communication between them is usually bizarre and unsatisfying. When, as part of the SAGE Project, we first began leading groups in these homes, I was frustrated by the difficulty I experienced in communicating with these people, who would only stare at me out of glassy, lifeless eyes. Yet as the weeks passed and they became more comfortable with my presence, I noticed that many of them slowly became more able to hear me when I spoke and more able to respond when I led exercises. After several months, nearly all the people who had initially been hard of hearing were able to respond appropriately and intelligently to the activities in the groups. In many cases, the so-called senility began to evaporate slowly as well.

It was frightfully clear to all of us involved in this work that many of these people had made a conscious or unconscious decision that there was no longer any reason to hear others or to function socially. As a result, they had become hard of hearing and "senile." But through their SAGE experience, many of these people decided that there was something worth hearing, and that sharing and communicating with other people could still be a worthwhile and stimulating activity. Staff members in these senior residences were shocked to find that so many of these older people became able to dramatically redevelop their ability to hear.

In addition to being used for hearing, your ears also serve another vital bodymind function, for they contain the delicate semicircular canals that are responsible for maintaining a sense of balance within your bodymind. These canals are filled with fluid, and as you move, the fluid in the canals also moves, continually telling your brain where up is and where down is. When you disturb the functioning of these canals, you lose your sense of equilibrium and, correspondingly, your feeling of security in the world. We forget how dependent we are on these tiny structures for balance and self-control. But if dis-ease or psychoemotional stress impairs their healthy functioning, we quickly appreciate the important role that they play in keeping us upright and centered.

THE EYES

Another psychosomatically important region is that which includes and surrounds the eyes. According to Elsworth Baker, armoring in this region "consists of a contraction and immobilization of the greater part of all of the muscles around the eye, eyelids, forehead, and tear glands, as well as the deep muscles at the base of the occiput—involving even the brain itself."[5]

To a large extent, the eyes reflect the health or dis-ease of the bodymind, and one can explore these manifestations in a number of ways: by noting the characteristic expression of the eyes and their placement in the sockets; by observing the actual structure and functioning of the eyeball itself; and by examining the condition of the iris and sclera.

What do your eyes reveal about your inner feelings, your passions, your fears? In what way are your eyes truly "windows to your soul"? You might put this book down a minute and go look at your eyes in a mirror. When you look at them, try to see them as though for the first time. As soon as you see their reflection in the mirror, look away for a moment and try to get a sense of what your eyes express nonverbally about you. Then look back into the mirror and examine your eyes in terms of their shape, their brightness, the way in which they rest in your face.

Eye Shapes

To illustrate some of the ways in which the eyes reflect the inner person, I will describe several different types of eyes and share with you what I believe they indicate.

Large, round eyes frequently reflect a warm, loving personality. This basic type of eye structure projects a caring attitude, as though the person were softly reaching out with his eyes to make honest and loving contact. Large, rounded eyes usually make other people feel comfortable in their presence.

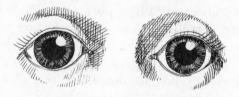

9-1. Large, Round Eyes

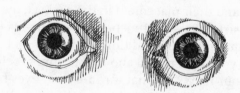

9-2. Bulging Eyes

Bulging eyes, on the other hand, indicate a nervous, penetrating way of being in the world. Such a person will, in a sense, be forcefully reaching out with his eyes and will often make other people uncomfortable and anxious in his presence. As a result, the eyes will usually discourage rather than attract warm feelings from other people.

Eyes that are deeply set within the eye sockets often indicate a lifetime of withheld expressions and withdrawn sadness. It is as though, in an attempt to guard and protect himself, this person has tried to pull his eyes and their seeing powers inward to his core. Deep-set eyes also frequently indicate that the person spends a large amount of time critically observing the actions and activities of others. From their receded position, the eyes seem to methodically absorb information like the lens of a camera.

I have worked with people who have what I call *"baby eyes."* These eyes are characterized by a wide-open, pleading quality and often belong to people who were Mamma's

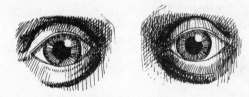

9-3. Deep-Set Eyes

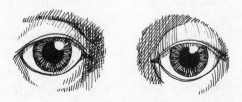

9-4. "Baby Eyes"

little boys or Daddy's little girls. Baby eyes are doubly expressive. First, they may show that the person has not allowed the ocular segment of his face to mature and develop fully. Second, baby eyes usually turn out to be extremely seductive and manipulative. This individual may be using his soft and sensual eyes to hold you while he attempts to draw you closer to him. I am not saying that these attributes or activities are necessarily negative or harmful; rather, they seem to be related to a slightly immature way of seeing and being seen in the world.

There seems to be some correspondence between the hardness or softness of a person's eyes and his interpersonal relationships. In general, the individual with hard, tense eyes sees the world in terms of how he might control it. These eyes are overly aggressive and assertive and seem to reach out and grab whatever they are focusing on. On the other hand, eyes that appear soft reflect a passive, receptive way of seeing the world. The soft-eyed person will tend to be easygoing and relaxed, perhaps slightly less able or willing to control the activities of his own life than is his hard-eyed counterpart.

Nearsightedness and Farsightedness

Another dimension of the psychosomatic nature of the eyes has to do with nearsightedness and farsightedness. In general, I have observed that when people are myopic, or near-sighted, they may tend to have difficulty projecting themselves outward. In a sense, their interpersonal vision is comfortably focused more on "near" than on "far" activities. These people are often inwardly focused or shy and may also tend to be highly rational and introspective. Myopia can sometimes be traced to an early trauma in which the person experienced something that was so uncomfortable that it forced him to, in a sense, withdraw his sight, thereby affecting the future development of his eyeball. Some people believe that myopia is largely the result of traumatized eye muscles, and that when the trauma or conflict is resolved, the muscles of the eye are then freed to develop and form in a more natural, vital fashion.[6]

I recently had an opportunity to explore the psychosomatic nature of myopia with a woman who is in her late sixties and came to me complaining of severe eye difficulty as well as chronic tension in her chest. She had been diagnosed as myopic when she was a small child and had been wearing glasses ever since. In the past few years, she had developed cataracts on both her eyes and was struggling to discover ways to relieve the dis-ease that was accumulating in and around her eyes.

After working with her for several months in an attempt to improve her overall state of health and vitality with yoga, mild bioenergetics, and basic Gestalt work, I decided to delve more deeply into her psychosomatic ocular conditioning with a guided fantasy technique. I had her lie comfortably on a couch as I slowly began to monitor her breathing. With the help of my suggestions, she began to relax, and as she did, her body grew more limp and her breathing slowed down considerably. When I felt that she was sufficiently focused and relaxed, I asked her to try to get a visceral sense of the way that she held tension in her entire bodymind. With her eyes closed, she traveled inward through her body and quickly began to imagine the way she felt when she was either afraid or uptight. She reported to me that when she felt this way, her breathing grew shallow, her chest grew rigid, her solar plexus contracted, and her eyes tightened. I asked her to assume this bodymind attitude for a few moments as she continued to lie on the couch, so that I could see this exaggerated attitude more clearly and so that she could get a well-defined feeling sense of how she responded to such uncomfortable states. Next, after having her relax and release the image of tension, I asked her to allow her mind to wander until it happened upon the most recent instance in which she had felt this way in her entire bodymind. In a few moments, she reported that she had felt very tense and uncomfortable just a few nights before, while she was preparing dinner for several of her husband's friends. As she hurriedly organized the meal, she found herself worrying that it would not turn out very well and that her husband would be disappointed in her. As she cooked, she felt her shoulders and chest grow rigid and her eyes grow tight in their sockets—almost as though she wanted to hide within herself and not be seen on the outside. She said that she felt like the ostrich who, wanting to disappear, hides his head in the sand. She felt that she was doing this with her eyes in response to the pressure of the occasion. I then asked her to take a deep breath and to allow this image to disappear. As she relaxed once again, I asked her to let her mind wander a bit farther back in time and to see if she could locate another instance when she felt this way.

After a short while, she reported that she was back in 1960, in an evening class at the university, where she was trying to complete an exam paper. She was so nervous and worried that her thoughts froze, and she was unable to answer many of the questions. As she sat blankly in her classroom seat, she felt as though she wanted to run away and never be seen again, that she was a failure and that no one would be proud of her. She told me that her body felt almost concave, as though she were holding her chest and belly so tight as to make them arch inward. In addition, she said that she felt as though she were squeezing her eyes tight in an unsuccessful attempt to look inward for answers.

After having her release this image and relax, I then had her explore her even more distant history. She reported that she had traveled back to 1930, when she was nineteen years old, and had just arrived in New York from a small town in the Midwest. She told me that when she got there, she felt intellectually and socially inadequate; although she had been an outstanding student in her home town, she imagined that she would be a tragic failure in New York. She explained how looking for jobs and a place to live had scared her to her core and how she had felt that everyone could see right through her frailties and was laughing inside at her. In response, her breathing shallowed, her chest grew tight and sunken, and her eyes rigidified. Her attitude was one of chronic fear, and she said that she wanted to hide inside so that no one could bother or hurt her. As she related this memory to me, her eyes grew tight, and it appeared that she was trying to suck them inward, to protect them, her, from the harshness of the world.

Slowly we traveled back, from image to image, fearful situation to fearful situation. In each case the instances that she recalled were similar: she repeatedly found herself in a frightening and potentially threatening situation; she felt inadequate and thought that others would either make fun of her or be disappointed in her. In response, she held tightly to herself by drawing in the muscles of her chest and abdomen and especially by squeezing her eyes tight in an attempt to look inside for safety.

Eventually, her images took us to 1915, when she was four years old. Here, she recalled that her mother had just given birth to her younger brother. As she watched her mother fondle and caress the infant, she grew deeply sad and hurt. Feeling that her mother didn't love her any more, she began to retreat deep into her core, withdrawing consciousness from her eyes and chest. I asked her to assume the bodymind attitude that she might have been feeling at that time, and she shifted her position until she was tightly curled up in a self-protective ball on the couch. Her breathing was shallow and her body was tightly held, and it seemed as though she would squeeze her eyeballs right into the center of her head. She said she felt that she had disappointed her mother and that her mother had replaced her with another child. She was ashamed of herself for being such a failure and felt incredibly hurt at being rejected and abandoned. Yet, because of her self-perceived inadequacy as a human being, she felt that she had no right to ask for love and support. Instead, she assumed a chronically rigid attitude of frightened determination and attempted to get through her tasks—her life—all the while wanting to withdraw and hide within herself. Through all her images, the bodymind expression of tightly covered eyes and frozen chest was significantly present.

I then asked her what she would like to have had happen as that four-year-old child, and she at once said that she wanted me to hold and stroke her and that she also wanted to be able to cry, which apparently was difficult for her. Her tears began as soon as my hand touched her shoulder and continued for nearly fifteen minutes. It was as though she had been wanting to cry and to be appreciated all her life, and had assumed her particular bodymind attitude in response to her belief that she was not worthy. After she finished crying and returned her attention to the present, we talked for quite a while about how her emotional history had probably come to affect her present health conditions. It was obvious to us that her continual need to hide within herself had contributed to her myopia and to the newly developing cataracts. In addition, she offered the observation that the concave-chest feeling which she had felt and reported to me during her remembered moments of panic had gotten built into her everyday structure, for her chest muscles were, in fact, contracted, and she suffered quite regularly from chest-centered ailments such as bronchitis and chest colds.

The way in which this woman had come to draw in her sight as a result of her fears of being rejected, unloved, and unappreciated were all too clear in her self-constructed images. The insight that both of us gained about her particular form of psychosomatic nearsightedness has proved invaluable in determining ways in which she will need to redevelop her own sense of self before she will be willing to release the long-held tension in her eyes. While all myopic people do not share the exact same fears and conflicts as this woman, the general fear of self-extension is quite common among them. It indicates a way of seeing in which only that which is close up is comfortably embraced, while things that are at a distance from oneself are viewed as unclear, unknown, and a bit frightening.

A contrary condition, hyperopia, or farsightedness, often corresponds to an inability to perceive activities that occur up close. As a result, the farsighted person may find more psychosomatic comfort in involving himself with activities that keep his attention focused away from himself and looking outward. The individual with a hyperopic condition will tend to be extroverted and outgoing and probably not very introspective. Whereas the nearsighted person withdraws into himself for safety, the farsighted person seems to extend himself into activities and relationships and future-oriented thinking as a way to avoid having to engage and develop his inner self. And whereas the nearsighted person needs to learn to extend himself more comfortably into the world, the farsighted person would do well to withdraw himself a bit from the world and spend more time within himself in order to balance the particular bodymind weakness that is indicated by his eye condition.[7]

Another fascinating psychosomatic aspect of the eyes is that they seem to be not only "windows into the soul" but also windows into one's medical history. There are two interesting fields of bodymind diagnosis that rely heavily on the structure and coloration of the eyes as a way to diagnose the relative health or dis-ease of the entire bodymind. They are called iris diagnosis, or iridology, and sclera diagnosis, or sclerology. According to Dr. Bernard Jensen:

> By way of definition, iridology is a science whereby the doctor or operator can tell from the markings or signs in the

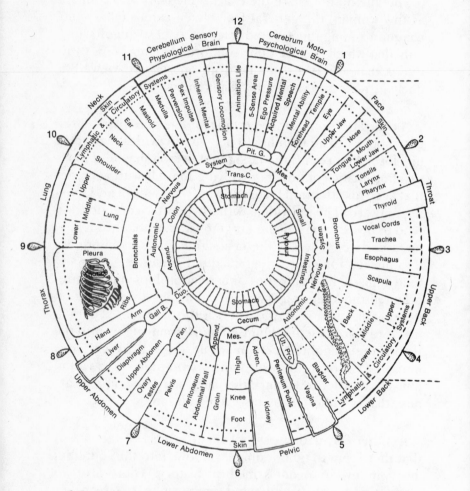

9-5. *Iris Diagnosis Chart: Right Eye (conceived by Dr. Bernard Jensen and drawn by Juan Barberis. Chart Copyright © 1977 by Dr. Bernard Jensen.)*

iris of the eye the reflex condition of the various organs of the body. In other words, it is the science of determining acute, sub-acute, chronic and destructive stages on the affected organs of the body through their corresponding

LEFT EYE

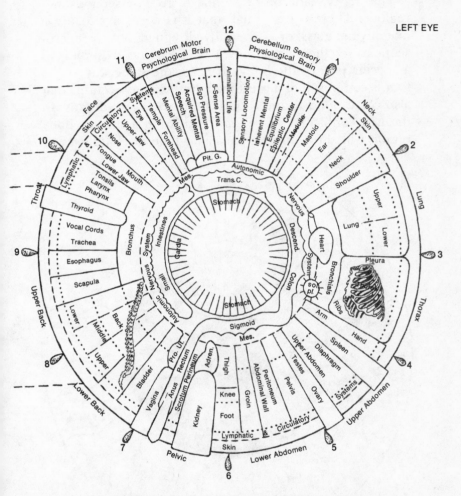

9-6. *Iris Diagnosis Chart: Left Eye (conceived by Dr. Bernard Jensen and drawn by Juan Barberis. Chart Copyright © 1977 by Dr. Bernard Jensen.)*

areas in the iris. Drug deposits, inherent weaknesses and living habits of the patient are also revealed in the iris of the eye.[8]

The iris is made up of a great many tiny sections and regions. These are so small that it is necessary to use a magnifying glass or a specially designed optical microscope to see them accurately. Each section corresponds to a specific part of the body, in much the same way as the foot is composed of a great many reflexology sections that also correspond to the various body parts and organs. In the iris, conflict, dis-ease, and toxicity in a specific body region will show up as a particular type of cloudiness or

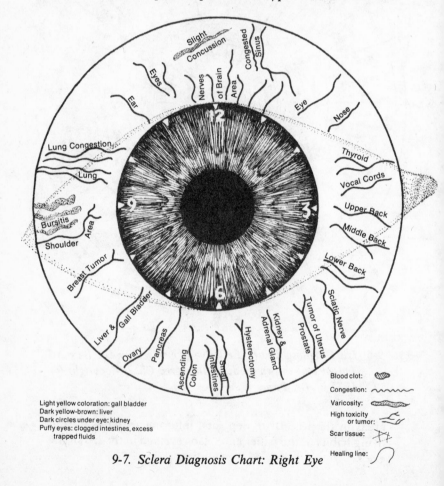

Light yellow coloration: gall bladder
Dark yellow-brown: liver
Dark circles under eye: kidney
Puffy eyes: clogged intestines, excess
    trapped fluids

Blood clot:
Congestion:
Varicosity:
High toxicity
or tumor:
Scar tissue:
Healing line:

9-7. Sclera Diagnosis Chart: Right Eye

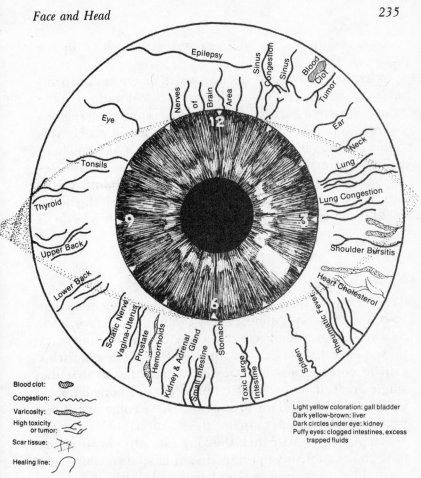

Blood clot:
Congestion:
Varicosity:
High toxicity or tumor:
Scar tissue:
Healing line:

Light yellow coloration: gall bladder
Dark yellow-brown: liver
Dark circles under eye: kidney
Puffy eyes: clogged intestines, excess
    trapped fluids

9-8. Sclera Diagnosis Chart: Left Eye

discoloration in the related iris section. Therefore, by examining the iris very closely and comparing its coloration to the iridology chart, you can learn a great deal about the health and well-being of an individual. People who are highly skilled in using the iris as a diagnostic map are sometimes able to detect regions in the body that are unwell even before the disease has surfaced and become noticeable. Other research in the field of iris diagnosis explains how various colorations of the eye reveal specific imbalances, toxicities, and weaknesses elsewhere in the body.

Sclerology is a similar science, which diagnoses the overall body state by reading the lines and discolorations of the sclera, the white portion of the eye. One notes what regions of the sclera are discolored or bloodshot and checks this information against a sclera diagnosis chart. Once you have gained information about internal conflicts and weaknesses of the bodymind through either of these diagnostic methods, you can then proceed to heal them through the bodymind technique or process that seems most appropriate to you.[9]

THE FOREHEAD

The muscles of the brow and forehead region are exercised in conjunction with almost every motion of the face, and, as a result, they tend to exhibit any chronic feelings and movements that we express with our faces. These muscles can be come easily overstressed. I have found that the single greatest contributor to tension in this bodymind region is thinking, and for this reason I have come to call the brow and forehead muscles the "rationality" muscles. When people overuse their thinking capacities or superimpose their rationality upon their spontaneous feelings and excitations, these muscles can become armored and tense.

For example, the woman who is helping with the editing of this book told me that when she spends large amounts of time reading and editing, she accumulates a great deal of tension in her forehead, which sometimes even leads to headaches. I watched her as she read my manuscript, and I noticed that as she read, she unconsciously furrowed her brow in an attitude that expressed diligence and intense concentration. I mentioned to her that by doing this she was working toward severely armoring the frontalis muscles in her forehead, and that this was obviously a contributing factor to her forehead tension and headaches.

She was surprised to hear that she had been doing this, but it immediately made sense to her; by heavily overusing these muscles in her intense intellectual activity, she was failing to allow her forehead the rest and relaxation time that it obviously needed. She seemed pleased with this realization and commented that she would try to spend more time in activities that incorporated the rest of her body, thus giving her "thinking muscles" a rest.

Tension and tension headaches in the region of the forehead may indicate that the person has been suppressing feelings with thought and exaggerated rationality. When this happens, the pressure of the unreleased emotions can build up in the top of the head, in very much the same way as carbonation becomes congested at the top of a soda bottle. When emotions are thus held down, they also can become distorted and wind up transforming themselves into feelings of anger, regardless of what they were to begin with. When people complain to me of headaches in his bodymind region, I often ask them who or what they are angry with. As soon as I say this, they usually smile and ask me, "How did you know?" If the emotions have been held down long enough to be transformed into anger and rage, I try to provide a therapeutic opportunity for the person to vent the rage and "blow his top" through appropriate psychoemotional exercises that might encourage yelling, complaining, biting, or crying. When the bottled-up emotions are freed in this fashion, tension in the forehead is usually lessened and many headaches immediately disappear.

A variety of personality traits and attitudes can be read from the lines and forms of this area. According to Alexander Lowen, for example, "a high brow denotes a person of refinement and intellectuality. Its opposite, the low brow, is a coarse fellow. A person is browbeaten when he looks downcast as a result of being intimidated by another's overbearing words or looks. His brows actually droop."[10] A tight-knitted brow usually reflects an intense, highly focused way of being in the world, whereas brows that nervously move up and down reflect a continual state of anxious surprise and lack of intellectual focus.

One of the easiest ways to explore the expressive nature of your brow and forehead is to sit in front of a mirror and make faces. As you try various facial posturings, first make the face with closed eyes and see how you feel internally when you hold yourself in this fashion. Then, open your eyes and try to sense the attitude that the outward expression on your face conveys. After you have made a variety of exaggerated and unusual faces, return to point zero and take a look at your real face, and see what it is saying to you.[11]

THE THIRD EYE: "AJNA"

The ocular section of the face houses the sixth Kundalini chakra, "Ajna," which is located between and a little above the brows. While this energy vortex is only one of the seven consciousness centers in the bodymind, it is the one that many of us relate to most intimately, for it corresponds to the development of heightened self-awareness and the expansion of mental powers.[12] Since many of us identify more closely with our mind than with any other aspect of ourselves, we tend to believe that the region of the third eye is, in fact, where our inner selves live, for our powers of reason and thought do generate from this crucial bodymind location.

Yet, as I have pointed out throughout this book, there are many ways that we can perceive the world other than with our intellects, and many ways that we can experience ourselves in addition to thinking.[13] In fact, all of the chakra regions represent modes of perception and awareness that we can make vital use of throughout our lives. As a result,

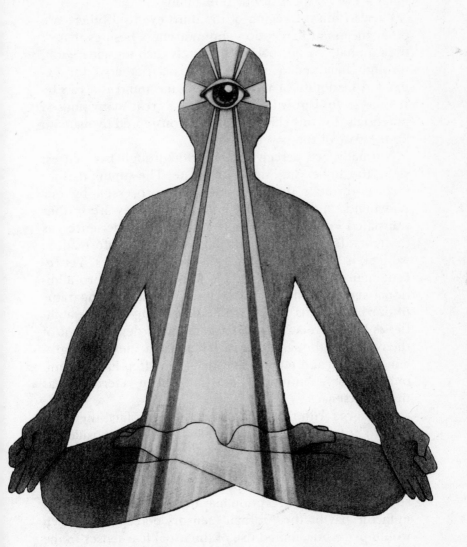

9-9. Sixth Chakra: Brow or Frontal Chakra

our selves, to the degree that they are alive and conscious, inhabit every aspect of our bodyminds.

Even within the region of the third eye itself, there are other means of perception and awareness besides that of the rational, intellectual mind. Just as each muscle region, through heightened awareness, has a potential for expanded flexibility of movement, so the mind too can be seen as a domain within which live a great many unused potentials, for this chakra region is considered by many to be the seat of the psychic senses.

Normally, we perceive the world through five senses: sight, touch, hearing, smell, and taste. The stimuli that we receive through these channels are processed by our bodyminds and sent to the brain, where they are further translated into information that we experience as thoughts, feelings, and perceptions, and this information, we feel, is all that we receive through our senses. Yet recent neurological research suggests that there are additional senses available to us within the natural apparatus of our bodyminds, and that the uncovering of these abilities is largely related to the opening and development of the region of the sixth chakra. These capacities for heightened psychic and mental sensitivity are often lumped into one category, "intuition," and have been referred to as the sixth sense.

I disagree with this categorization, for in fact, there appear to be *seven* psychic senses, in addition to the usual five senses, through which the human bodymind is capable of perception. Perception through these senses is usually referred to as "extrasensory perception" and I would like to suggest that such perception may not be "extra" at all, that in fact it may be the "normal" sensory perception—which would place our limited use of the usual five senses in the category of "deficient" sensory perception. The seven psychic senses which have been distinguished (there might very well be more undiscovered senses) are:

1. Telepathy—the ability to communicate with another mind without the use of any of the basic five senses.

2. Precognition or future access—the ability to perceive information across time into the future.

3. Retrocognition or past access—the ability to perceive previous events and information back through time.

4. Clairvoyance—the ability to perceive situations and information at a distance directly, without the mediation of another mind or article.

5. Vibrational empathy—the ability to accomplish such sensory activities as divining, reading auras, astral traveling, healing, and locating lost objects.

6. Psychometry—the ability to touch something and sense its relationship to people, time, etc., entirely through contact with this object.

7. Psychokinesis—the ability to influence the nature of physical matter without any physical contact, purely with the powers of the mind.

It is not within the scope of this book to elaborate any more fully upon the varieties of psychic experience or upon the particular arguments that surround such discussions. Yet I would like to emphasize my belief that the realization of psychic or extrasensory abilities is not something necessarily magical or mystical. Rather, as is the case with all human abilities and potentialities, these talents are among the vastly unused powers that live within the normal human bodymind, awaiting discovery.[14]

Whether we are aware of our psychic senses or not, it is clear to me that we are making use of only a portion of the powers of mind and self-consciousness that seem to live within the domain of the sixth chakra. Once again, I believe the reason we are only partly alive in this vital bodymind region is that we have developed certain ways of perceiving, thinking, and imaging which, while highly functional, also tend to limit our more expansive visions and thoughts. As we surely limit our range of physical movement by rigidifying and armoring our musculature, so might we also limit our mental powers by armoring them with fears, intellectual conflicts, and contractive beliefs.

In order to keep ourselves functioning within the comfortable structures of our lives, cultures, and personal beliefs, we tend to use our brains and nervous systems primarily to sort out and eliminate information that would otherwise overpower us with its force in much the same way as unarmored musculature might overwhelm us with its electric feelings of life and expansiveness. In fact, Aldous Huxley goes so far as to suggest that for most of us "the function of the brain and nervous system is to protect us from being overwhelmed and confused by this mass of largely useless and irrelevant knowledge, by shutting out most of what we should otherwise perceive or remember at any moment, and leaving only that very small selection which is likely to be practically useful."[15] Because we need to limit the degree to which we are experiencing the full pulsation and force of the universe, we stop ourselves from being aware of a great many of our mental powers, such as the psychic senses. As a result, our conception of ourselves and of the universe is derived through partially closed receptors, which, in turn, keep us from seeing past our limitations.

Yet, when we have explored and developed enough of ourselves to have reached a stage of personal development that corresponds to the level of the sixth chakra, we are more able and prepared to experience ourselves fully and consciously. As our bodyminds become more free of tension, conflict, and self-limiting fears, we begin to allow ourselves a larger, more expansive insight into ourselves and into the universe of which we are a part. In fact, the more open we become in our ability to be truly alive, the more full, alive, and interconnected everything else seems. At this level of development, there is a strong and vibrant recognition of the unity of all things as the tensions and barriers that usually limit and separate them dissolve.

Since the inner qualities of the third-eye chakra are concerned with the development of the heightened self-awareness that comes when muscular armor is released, psychoemotional armor dissolved, and mental limitations expanded, I have decided that the most appropriate way for me to continue an exploration of this topic is to include it in a discussion of the human-potential movement and some of the ways in which the various "growth" techniques allow us to become more self-aware and less self-restrictive.

SELF-DEVELOPMENT

In the past few years, hundreds of thousands of relatively healthy, happy people have begun to explore themselves through some aspect of the rapidly expanding human-potential movement. A businessman from New York City meditates twice each day, silently reciting the mantra that his transcendental-meditation checker selected for him. A U.S. Forest Service employee in Montgomery, Alabama, jogs three miles each day during his lunch break. A housewife in Denver experiences ten Rolfing sessions and discovers that they have made her feel considerably healthier. High school students in Chicago take a course in sensitivity training designed to enhance their interest in education. A widowed grandmother in Washington, D.C., signs up for the two EST training weekends. A policeman in Miami has begun to practice yoga each morning before he goes out on his daily rounds. Psychiatrists in Philadelphia study the Feldenkrais method for bodymind development and begin to incorporate these exercises into the regular activities at their community health clinic. A minister in Seattle undergoes bioenergetic therapy twice each week and begins to discover the love and compassion that live within his armored body. Representatives from the navy meet in Big Sur, California, for an intensive week of encounter and sensory awareness. Senior citizens in Eugene, Oregon, learn to control their own blood pressure with biofeedback training.

The human-potential movement and its various approaches and techniques seem to be spreading throughout the country, affecting larger and larger numbers of people. Beginning as an almost mystical cult, with several thousand die-hard participants, most of them middle-class and highly educated, it has finally begun to expand and fortify itself by branching out into a variety of health, educational, business, and religious institutions, across a wide range of social and economic groups. Wellness and personal growth seem to be on a lot of people's minds these days.

Why are so many people expending the time, energy, and money to study these self-development techniques? Why are people from all over the country, from all walks of life, beginning to engage in self-exploration? Why has there lately been a sudden upsurge of interest in consciousness, awareness, and human potential?

If you were to question people who engage in these activities about why they do so, most would probably answer, "It makes me feel better," or, "I'm curious to learn more about myself." While these responses seem absurdly simplistic they nevertheless profoundly reflect the basic fact that many of us are looking for ways to counteract the tension and stress that accompany twentieth-century living while simultaneously enhancing the quality and quantity of pleasure, health, creativity, and happiness of our own lives. In order to feel better and to gain greater self-knowledge, many people have begun to take part in methods and techniques specifically designed to promote the feelings of well-being, tension release, and increased self-responsibility that so many of our other activities work directly against.

While the approaches are different and, indeed, sometimes contradictory, most share the goal of providing vehicles through which we can all learn to explore, expand, and develop our human capabilities and potentialities. By educating ourselves about our own strengths and weaknesses, we can begin to teach ourselves how to increase our chances of experiencing health and peace of mind, and simultaneously decrease the likelihood of stress and unhappiness. With the advent of the growth movement, therapeutic education for the masses becomes a reality, as the traditional roles of doctor, minister, and "shrink" are slowly replaced by the guru, guide, and "stretch." Psychology, psychiatry, self-reflection, change, and self-improvement are no longer just for the sick or unhappy but are becoming available in shorthand form for healthy people as well.[16]

This movement toward super-health, greater self-knowledge, and happiness by an ever-increasing number of people is more than just a narcissistic escape from the harsh realities and stress of twentieth-century living. Rather, it seems to me that underlying much of the interest in growth and self-development is a sincere desire to improve the human condition by acknowledging and then initiating the attitudes, feelings, and activities that influence its positive development.

To illustrate this point, I would like to spend a few moments examining the recent attraction to meditation here in the United States. Since the meditation bug has bitten everyone from spiritual aspirants seeking enlightenment to nervous business executives looking for ways to get more for their money, it holds special interest to me as a popular human-potential technique. By spending some time examining the nature of meditation, I hope to perform two functions: first, I will share with you some of my own beliefs and experiences in regard to this much-practiced, highly controversial activity; and, second, using meditation as an example, I will illustrate some of the relationships that I see between the techniques of growth and the true feelings of growth and personal development.

Meditation

For me, meditation is simply a *word*. It is a word that describes a particular mood or state of consciousness that your bodymind enters at certain times throughout your life. This mood, or feeling state, usually occurs when you are totally and selflessly involved in an activity to the point that there is little or no separation between you and what you are doing. At this moment, you are so absorbed in simply "being" that your consciousness becomes tightly focused on the activity at hand, most of your usual mental chatter ceases, physical distraction and stress diminish, and the passage of time seems to be irrelevant.[17]

Before I proceed with my discussion, you might like to think for a few moments about the times when you have felt this way and about what you were engaged in at those times.

As you may have realized, the feeling state that is described by the word meditation can occur at nearly any time. For example, you may have felt this way while you were making love last night. When you lovingly joined with your partner, you may have found that your thoughts quieted down and that your feelings rose and consumed you with their fullness and passion. During these moments of selfless communion, you probably lost track of all your usual worries and bodymind distractions and gave yourself over to the power and simplicity of the situation.

Or perhaps you experience meditation as you carefully prune the roses in your garden. As you deeply immerse yourself in the process of working with the roses, the rest of the world seems to drift away, allowing time to disappear temporarily and leaving you with a mood or emotional state characterized by warm, clear feelings and perceptions.

You might meditate while playing the flute. As you gently breathe into the mouthpiece of the instrument, translating air into melody, all distraction ceases and you feel a kind of oneness with your instrument. At this point, your body-mind is deeply and effortlessly at one with itself, aided by the instrument on which you are focusing.

Or the meditative feeling might enfold you as you sit alone before your fireplace on a chilly winter evening. As the flames swirl and dance, you become hypnotized by their fury and fancy. For a while, you become the fire itself, as the separation between you and it disappears. The clarity and warmth of the contact is felt in every cell of your body-mind. It's as though the focus the fire presents to you, with its curious changes and evolving radiance, allows you to step outside yourself for a bit, leaving behind all the mental chatter and physical tension that normally influence your thoughts, feelings, and perceptions. During these rare moments of ecstasy, you have transcended your usual self; there is no longer any separation between you, the perceiver, and that which is being perceived. All there is, is "now," and you find yourself fully and actively engaged in its flow.

These moments can and do occur to different people at different times. While the factors that give birth to the meditative experience can be surprisingly varied, the feelings that characterize the state are relatively similar and consistent among most people. And while the meditative experience does not lend itself very well to verbal description, words and phrases like *peaceful, relaxed, beautiful, peace of mind, lack of tension, transcendent, simple, out of the ordinary, selfless, union, spiritual, with the flow,* and *timeless* are frequently used to describe this state of consciousness.

Meditation, then, is a word that describes a state of consciousness, a mood, an attitude, a feeling tone. It is *not* the

physical location where this feeling emerged, nor is it the
position the body was in during the meditation, nor is it the
clothing you wore while you felt this way. This point is well
captured by Joel Kramer:

> Real meditation is not something one does for five minutes
> or fifteen minutes, sitting in the most uncomfortable posi-
> tion one can possibly get into because the more pain I feel
> the more righteous I am. Real meditation is watching so that
> there is no separation between the watcher and the
> watched. It involves a quality of attention that has to do with
> seeing what is. Meditation is not a removal from the world.
> Real meditation is not simply a passive thing; it's an extraor-
> dinary activity, an activity without effort that involves a di-
> rect confrontation with that which is, always containing
> within it the eternal.[18]

This state of presence and selflessness is usually accompanied by increased feelings of clarity and peace of mind,
decreased bodymind stress, and heightened awareness.

When these moments occur, we do not usually perceive
them at once with our rational minds; if we were to evaluate
our experience intellectually, we would probably disperse
the state by which the experience is defined. Feelings of
clarity and selflessness are elusive butterflies; once you try
to catch them with thoughts and pin them down with
words, they immediately fly away or wither. The reflection
and evaluation usually come later on, with "That was very
beautiful," or "I sure feel wonderful," or "That was the
most peaceful experience I have ever had."

Meditative experiences are usually profoundly enjoyable
and nourishing, for they allow us to get in touch with the
feelings of clarity and happiness that live within us, buried
deep beneath layers of stress, armor, and ego. Abraham
Maslow called moments like these "peak experiences,"[19]
and suggested that they serve a vital human function in that
they allow us to take brief journeys out of our usual body-

mind state into realms of feeling and consciousness that are, in a sense, transcendent. Maslow felt that peak experiences pull us upward by our bootstraps, bringing us to a more aware, more alive, more creative way of being.

Now, when I have had an experience that felt great, I will probably try to have it again. However, I have been brought up with the silly notion that pleasure can be packaged and duplicated, so a part of me has come to believe that when I feel good, it is because of a place where I am physically located, or because of the specific people I am with or the clothing I am wearing. I am discovering, however, that the meditative experience seems to be more dependent on my own inner state of development and receptivity than it is on any outside or external factors.

For example, if I had a "peak experience" one sunny afternoon on a beach in the Virgin Islands, I might associate my pleasant feelings of that day with that particular beach and dream of returning there for a similar experience. Or if I reached this meditative state while making love one night and now my lover has left me, I might try to find her again so as to re-create the wonderful moments of loving ecstasy that have imprinted themselves on my bodymind memory.

Yet the nature of these experiences is that they are terribly difficult to re-create and even more difficult to repeat in the same form. While many environments are surely conducive to enjoyable feelings, trying to restage one such time or place tends to stifle the spontaneity and innocence that very probably characterized the splendor of the initial experience.

Yet if I felt so good during those moments, how can I learn to feel that way again? Who or what can teach me to get back into that relaxed, selfless state of bodymind peace and harmony?

Apparently, people have been asking these questions throughout history, and in response, a variety of meditative techniques have emerged. Here in the United States, a number of them have become familiar to large groups of people. With names like transcendental meditation, Rajneesh meditation, Vipassasa meditation, mantric meditation, zazen meditation, yoga meditation, and T'ai Chi meditation, these practices have emerged to allow us to learn how to quiet our minds, relax our emotions, improve our overall bodymind states of being, and explore our inner selves. Each of these meditative approaches to personal growth has attempted to isolate several of the characteristics of happiness, health, and peace of mind from the entire spectrum of human experience and has developed specific exercises and activities designed to heighten self-awareness and increase the probability of the recurrence of these desired feelings.

For example, I have discovered that my mind tends to quiet down considerably if I sit comfortably erect and allow myself to step aside from my usual thoughts and distractions in "zazen" fashion. If I am pleased with the way I feel when my mind relaxes in this fashion, I might begin to practice mind-quieting exercises regularly in order to sustain the mellow and aware feelings generated by such exercises. The more I participate in this type of activity, the more relaxed and self-aware I become.

Perhaps the different meditative techniques have emerged in order to take the randomness out of emotional experience and to create and sustain pleasurable, nourishing, and enlightening feelings. By developing techniques that have a high probability of reproducing the internal feelings and states that spontaneously emerge in those rare moments of existential clarity, mankind has been cultivating a kind of human software technology, designed to educate people to get in tune with the desired feelings and to begin to build them into everyday living patterns.

Before I continue with my discussion, I want to re-emphasize the fact that these meditative techniques are only vehicles through which you may learn to explore and develop yourself; the techniques themselves are not the meditative feelings, nor are they the states of consciousness.

For example, several years ago I took a course in meditation with a well-known meditation teacher. I have been meditating on and off for eight years, yet I was curious to experience the way this individual would present this elusive topic. The class was called "Introduction to Meditation" and was filled with people of all shapes, sizes, and costumes. I also took the course because I wanted to learn to relax more fully and to quiet the intellectual chatter that usually fills up my mind.

Each week, nearly one hundred of us took our seats, cross-legged, on small meditation cushions that were placed on the floor in a beautifully adorned meditation room. Our meditation teacher sat before us on a simple cushion, explaining to our eager ears how meditation was a simple process, one that would allow us to relax our bodyminds and move us into higher states of consciousness.

Well, each night as we began our sitting meditational exercises, I did, in fact, quickly move to another state of consciousness—sleep. No matter how hard I tried, I was simply not comfortable sitting cross-legged on a tiny cushion trying to force myself to feel blissful. No doubt that was my problem: trying too hard. But I have decided that it's all right to fail in at least half my human-potential explorations, so I have chalked my meditation class up to experience. For me this was another example of how a wrapper is still only a wrapper, no matter how curious it is, and of how the *real* item apparently waits within, independent of its outer coverings.

Thus, sitting in the lotus position for an hour does not ensure an altered state of consciousness. Similarly, practicing the flute does not ensure that you will learn how to play it. Yet, in all fairness, many of the meditative techniques do seem to be highly developed and reliably workable practices that effectively allow large numbers of people to learn to isolate some of the factors that contribute to states of health, peace of mind, and overall well-being. Actively engaging in these exercises, you can increase the probability of the continued occurrence of these states. While the practicing does not ensure the finished product, many techniques surely do seem to raise the odds on its emergence.

As I see it, the widespread use of meditative exercises has two fascinating aspects. First, these exercises allow us the opportunity to personally and experientially discover that there are a number of different moods, attitudes, and states of consciousness that can be entered into and experienced besides the everyday state of chronic low-grade stress that characterizes many of our lives. These meditative techniques and exercises are a powerful tool for observing and exploring our internal bodymind processes, thereby leaving us considerably more self-aware and more able to map our inner and outer bodymind terrains.

The second interesting aspect of the use of the meditative exercises is that in addition to enabling us to become more aware of our states of consciousness, they also allow us to learn to influence and control these moods, feelings, and bodymind conditions, leaving us more responsible for our own lives and evolutions. By learning to increase the probability of desired moods and feelings through heightened self-awareness and creative self-regulation, while simultaneously decreasing the occurrence of the negative states of ill health and psychoemotional anxiety, we begin to exercise more fully our uniquely human powers of self-reflective and self-aware action. I believe that the widespread use of the meditative techniques is one factor in the emergence of a new set of beliefs about the degree to which we can consciously affect or influence our feelings, creativity, and state of health or ill health. By learning to be aware of ourselves and of the vast powers of our bodyminds, we are gradually becoming more in control of our human potentialities and, by so doing, are slowly but surely taking another giant step along the path of our own evolution.

Human-Potential Techniques

The lessons learned about human self-education through the examination of meditative techniques can be generalized across a wider range of human-potential processes and activities. For yoga, T'ai Chi, Rolfing, bioenergetics, Reichian energetics, the Feldenkrais method, meditation, Gestalt therapy, biofeedback, and most forms of exercise at their most basic level are simply other experiential processes designed to allow us to become more constructively aware of ourselves. What is most important about these techniques is their emphasis on direct personal experience and on self-initiated change and self-improvement. Once again, encounter and bioenergetic therapy are not necessarily, in themselves, desirable activities (although I know people who eat them like candy). Rather, it is the way you feel and what you can learn about yourself when you engage in them that is important.

I have come to see that all these human-potential processes are a bit like existential fun-house mirrors, each of which has a slight distortion to it yet is nevertheless able to reveal a particular image of me to myself. By approaching my personal growth from this viewpoint, I have become able to befriend many of my previously undiscovered or mistreated bodymind strengths and weaknesses. By learning to see myself from a variety of angles and perspectives, I have placed myself in a position of greater honesty and intimacy in relation to myself, and it becomes increasingly easy for me to influence my own growth and development in a positive fashion.[20]

For example, through my experience with encounter therapy, I have learned to be more honest with myself and with others and more up front about my feelings and wishes. Because of this, I find that there is more clarity to my life and more integrity to my relationships. Through my Rolfing experience, I have learned both intellectually and physically how I hold myself and how I store tension as well as pleasure deep within my bodymind. With this increased self-knowledge, I have become more able to diminish my psychosomatic weaknesses with helpful exercise and mindfulness, while strengthening those parts of me that are already vital and alive. Similarly, meditative exercises have allowed me to see myself from an entirely different perspective. Through their regular practice I have learned to be more aware of the various feelings and emotional moods that make up my particular personality. With this awareness, I have become less manipulated by the chattering of my mind and more responsive to its creative drives. Each of these various processes and techniques has allowed me to learn more about myself so that I have become more self-aware and therefore more self-responsible. It is my belief that the more fully I know myself the more able I will be to lead a thoroughly nourishing, loving, and creative life.

While I obviously feel that many of the growth techniques and processes can help you to become more aware of your feelings and bodymind potentialities, I realize that they do not always lead to growth and enlightenment. In fact, I have met hundreds of people who, after having experienced many hours of yoga, biofeedback, or encounter, still seem to be exactly the same as they were before they began their "self-development" odyssey—except, of course, that now they have a new vocabulary.

Furthermore, any experience or activity that allows me to know myself more fully can legitimately be thought of as a "growth" process, whether it's listed in the Esalen catalogue or not. Growth and self-awareness are states of being, they are experiences, they are expressions of your own personal life development. As such, they are only partly related to the activities and techniques that have sprung up in their name.

These human-potential processes are simply techniques —noble techniques, but techniques nonetheless. Although they hold the potential for educating us about ourselves and teaching us to be healthy and happy, we must not forget what they are or begin to worship them or put them above our own experience. For me, the most upsetting aspect of the growth movement is that so many people have forgotten that the techniques and the gurus are there to encourage us to know and appreciate ourselves. Frequently we leave our classes and workshops appreciating the guru and his techniques while continuing to feel crummy about ourselves. When this happens, gurus and experiences become like trophies that one places on the mantel to let people know just how far one has come. Yet these collected trophies and experiences are only external signs and don't necessarily have a direct relationship to the level of development of their owner.

For me, the most wonderful aspect of the human-potential movement is that it has given birth to a legion of teachers and techniques that are capable of helping me learn more about myself. Depending on their particular focus, they can help me to see things about my body, my mind, my bodymind, my life, and my dreams. This increased self-awareness places me in a position where I come closer to becoming the master of my own life by developing myself in such a way as to enhance my strengths and creativities while diminishing my conflicts and fears.

It is here in my own personal growth, corresponding to the qualities and characteristics of the sixth Kundalini chakra, that I begin to really know myself in the fullest sense.

CHAPTER

BODYMIND

THROUGHOUT THIS BOOK, I have described how the body-mind develops tensions, blockages, and psychosomatic imbalances. I have suggested that there are ways the body-mind can be explored and developed, and relieved of many of the conflicts and limitations that thwart its further development. By descriptively ascending through the various regions of the bodymind, I have attempted to show how the habits and preferences of the mind are reflected in the shape and form of the body, and how each of the Kundalini chakras seems to relate not only to a part of the body but to a stage of human development as well.

When we reach the seventh chakra, it becomes all too clear that the territories of the first six chakras can be compared to obstacles and challenges along a path that one travels in order to approach the state of self-realization that corresponds to the awakening of this seventh, final chakra. The seventh Kundalini chakra, "Sahasrara," sits atop the head, crowning the entire bodymind, and connects to the

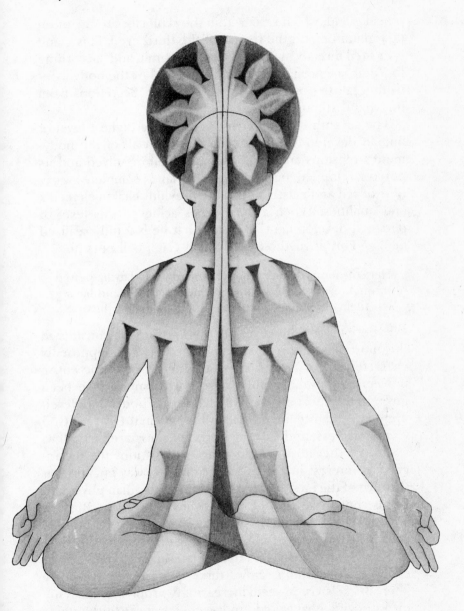

10-1. Seventh Chakra: Crown or Coronal Chakra

pineal gland, which rests within the skull close to the pituitary gland behind the region of the third eye.[1] This gland is located directly in the middle of the brain and "according to Yogic science . . . is the master gland of the body, controlling all the other glands of the body. Secretions from this gland stimulate all other glands."[2]

The seventh chakra corresponds to the highest level of human development, the point at which all of the bodymind's tensions and conflicts have been dissolved and its potentials tapped. Its attainment demands complete awareness of self and mastery of all the previous chakra elements and qualities. When a person has achieved this level of personal development, it is said that he is a fully realized being.[3] For, as mythologist Joseph Campbell puts it:

> Here the journey ends. The serpent goddess, having passed through every form of consciousness and life, and having left them all behind, has risen to her fullest height.[4]

Experience of this level of consciousness is considered the most blissful and beautiful of all and is supposedly characterized by a clear sense of oneness with the entire universe. Many beautifully descriptive names have been given to this most elevated of all levels of bodymind development: Enlightenment, Samadhi, Nirvana, Heaven, God Consciousness, and Cosmic Consciousness are just a few.

One of the most enlightening explanations for the increased interest in human consciousness was put forth at the turn of the nineteenth century by a Canadian physician. In his controversial book *Cosmic Consciousness,* Dr. Richard M. Bucke offered simple descriptions of the categories of consciousness, as well as a fascinating discussion of the way these levels of awareness might relate to one another in an evolutionary fashion. Now, three-quarters of a century later, Bucke's vision seem increasingly prophetic. In all my own studying I have not found a simpler, more to-the-point analysis of the evolution of human consciousness with which we are at present involved. For this reason, I have decided to incorporate some of Bucke's descriptions and ideas into this chapter on the seventh chakra and the evolutionary significance of self-realization.

Bucke felt that at some time in the twentieth century a point would come when the human race would make some sort of quantum leap in its own evolution to a condition of expansive self-awareness, greater intellectual clarity, higher consciousness, and loving unity among all beings of this earth. He felt this change would come about when sufficient information and experience had been generated to enable mankind to emerge from the conflicts, confusions, ignorances, and psychoemotional poverties within which it had become trapped by its own limitations and stressful developments.

Bucke suggested that this transformation would be focused upon exploration of the untapped domains of the body and mind, and that these developments would allow for the birth of a new and higher perspective, an elevated way of being, feeling, seeing, knowing, and relating. He felt that this evolutionary development would be aided by an emerging assortment of teachers, as well as by a corresponding collection of techniques, activities, and processes focused upon heightened awareness and the expansion of human knowledge. The outcome of this change process would be mankind's eventual evolution to a new level of human consciousness which he called "cosmic consciousness."

Our descendants will sooner or later reach, as a race, the condition of cosmic consciousness, just as, long ago, our ancestors passed from simple to self-consciousness. . . . This step in evolution is even now being made since it is clear . . . that men with this faculty in question are becoming more and more common and also that as a race we are approaching nearer to that stage of the self-conscious mind from which the transition to the cosmic conscious is effected.[5]

In explaining this possibile evolution of human awareness, Bucke identified three major gradations of consciousness. The first, most elemental level is that which he called "simple consciousness":

> . . . which is possessed by, say, the upper half of the animal kingdom. By means of this faculty a dog or a horse is just as conscious of the things about him as man is; he is also conscious of his own limbs and body and he knows that these are a part of himself.[6]

At this level of bodymind development, food, shelter, self-defense, and procreation are the primary life concerns and evolutionary motivations of the species. Yet past the basic capacities of simple consciousness exists another, more highly evolved dimension of awareness which Bucke called "self-consciousness":

> By virtue of this faculty man is not only conscious of trees, rocks, waters, his own limbs and body, but he becomes conscious of himself as a distinct entity apart from the rest of the universe.[7]

Since we are self-conscious beings, we simultaneously inhabit the worlds of sensations, perceptions, and biological urges as well as the world of language, beliefs, thought, and self-reflection. Stated simply, at this level of consciousness we are not only aware, we also know that we are aware.

A person who has fully developed his capacity for self-consciousness has mastered the qualities and challenges that characterize the first six chakras: survival, sexuality, power, love, communication, self-reflection, and self-awareness. Once this level of development has been achieved, he is now ready to explore and develop more fully the potential for wisdom and self-realization that live within the vast and splendid domain of the seventh chakra, the doorway to cosmic consciousness, which Bucke believed to be the ultimate level of human development.

With cosmic consciousness, simple and self-consciousness persist, but there is an added awareness of the unity of the cosmos and an integrated and deeply sensed feeling of connection to all its parts and processes. As Bucke states:

> The prime characteristic of cosmic consciousness is, as its name implies, a consciousness of the cosmos, that is, of the life and order of the universe. . . . There are many elements belonging to the cosmic sense besides the central fact just alluded to. Of these a few may be mentioned. Along with the consciousness of the cosmos there occurs an intellectual enlightenment or illumination which alone would place the individual on a new plane of existence—would make him almost a member of a new species. To this is added a state of moral exaltation, an indescribable feeling of elevation, elation, and joyousness, and a quickening of the moral sense, which is fully as striking and more important both to the individual and to the race than is the enhanced intellectual power. With these come what may be called a sense of immortality, a consciousness of eternal life, not a conviction that he shall have this, but the consciousness that he has it already.[8]

Bucke believed that human evolution to a state of cosmic consciousness would dramatically accelerate when large numbers of people became interested in exploring the realms and limitations of their own bodymind potentialities. This exploration would begin on a very private, personal level, but would eventually precipitate the development of a massive transformation of all human beliefs and forms.[9]

I strongly agree with Bucke that there does seem to be another, more elevated level of human consciousness beyond the borders of self-conscious existence, and that the evolutionary journey toward a state of cosmic consciousness may be upon us now. I do not feel that at this point in my own life I have achieved this state of awareness for more than fleeting moments, so I am unable to offer firsthand accounts of its nature. I have, however, seen enough evidence to believe that the recent worldwide interest in expanding bodymind potential and in cultivating techniques and processes that are designed to develop these powers indicates that self-reflection, self-improvement, and self-initiated change just might be the central channels through which this change in human awareness is beginning to occur.

The belief that self-development may be the process through which an evolutionary transformation to a higher state of human consciousness is developing can best be appreciated when we realize that we are at present the *end product* of the entire evolution of life on our planet. Having laboriously developed throughout hundreds of millions of years to our present state of being, we are, in a sense, riding on the crest of the evolutionary wave that has been pushing onward throughout history. This development has recorded itself in our bodyminds and, in addition, has molded our bodyminds into the vehicles, the human ships, by which this evolutionary journey is destined to continue.[10]

Therefore, with each passing moment, our bodyminds are in the process of flowing through time, carrying us from yesterday to tomorrow across a flexible bridge that is ourselves. In this way, all of our physical characteristics and shapes are acutely reflective of the physical and emotional activities of our lives, revealing our histories with their scars and uneven terrain, and also suggesting our futures with their potential for development and transformation.[11]

In this book, I have attempted to explore and discuss some of the ways we come to form and create ourselves with our experiences, habits, beliefs, and feelings. I have also tried to suggest that with bodymindfulness we can take greater responsibility for shaping futures that are free of conflict and dis-ease and filled with awareness and health. Since I believe that increased bodymind awareness can lead to greater self-knowledge and expanded potential, I have focused most of my discussion on the personal and psycho-physical factors of our lives to the exclusion of many of the cultural, hereditary, and nutritional components. By doing so, I have not meant to suggest that these other factors are unimportant, but rather that from my own experience I feel that the unanswered questions about the bodymind are most directly answered when approached in a direct and personal fashion.

At first brush, it might sound as if, by stressing my own need to explore and expand my bodymind limitations and horizons, I have been suggesting a totally self-centered, narcissistic approach to self-responsibility and planetary responsibility. This is far from true, however, for I believe that by working on myself I put myself in the most vital position to truly change and improve our social and cul-tural forms and flows. Since all my actions and interactions are extensions and projections of who I am, how I feel, and what I believe, the best I can do for others is to be my most open, creative, and loving "me." If I am unhappy, angry, or uptight within my self, all my actions and projections will be tinted and flavored with internal conflicts and limita-tions. When I am aware, open, and truly loving, all my activities, no matter how small or incidental, become ways in which I can serve the world in a loving and aware fashion and help to create it anew.

As I see it, the basic work has to be done at the starting point—on oneself. Social, cultural, and global interactions are dependent on the actions and movements of the in-dividuals who make up the physical and psychological net-work of the group. For the group to change and improve itself, its members must first change and develop.[12]

Some people feel that this is an entirely wrong way to pursue positive change, and that cultural rules, economic structures, and environmental conditions must first be altered before we can change. But what is the culture? What is the environment? What is economics? Aren't they merely our own constructions and projections? Aren't they just reflections of our own internal conflicts and possibilities? In order to alter our projections, we must first refocus the projector: *we must change ourselves.*

As I have repeatedly suggested throughout this book, I believe that the source of many of our conflicts lives within us, in our bodyminds. I also feel that in many instances, the resolution of these obstacles to growth and human development also lives within us, awaiting our exploration and discovery. I believe that the increasing interest in expanded awareness, wellness, and personal growth suggests that large numbers of people have become disenchanted with outward searching and dependence and have begun to look within for solutions and answers to the conflicts and diseases of their lives.

Since I view the bodymind as the evolutionary storehouse for all of life's potentials, I am hopeful that by exploring ourselves in this fashion and by attempting to develop more fully the various aspects and qualities of our bodyminds, we are steering ourselves into regions of greater self-knowledge within whose boundaries waits the embryonically developing transformation of human consciousness.

NOTES

Complete publishing information can be found in the Bibliography, pp. 279–291.

PREFACE

1. See Sheldon, Stevens, and Tucker, *The Varieties of Human Physique;* and Sheldon, *Atlas of Men.*
2. See Birdwhistell, *Kinesics and Context.*
3. See Wilhelm Reich, *Character Analysis.*
4. See Lowen, *The Language of the Body* and *Bioenergetics.*
5. See Alexander, *The Resurrection of the Body.*
6. See the Lomi Staff, *The Lomi Papers;* and Heckler, *The Mind/Body Interface.*
7. See Pesso, *Experience in Action.*
8. See Ichazo, *The Human Process for Enlightenment and Freedom.*
9. See Sweigard, *Human Movement Potential;* and Schoop and Mitchell, *Won't You Join The Dance?*

CHAPTER 1. BODY/MIND

1. For a description of the creation of bioenergetic therapy, see Lowen, *Bioenergetics.* Further explanations of bioenergetics can be obtained in the following books: Lowen, *The Betrayal of the Body, Depression and the Body, The Language of the Body, Love and Orgasm,* and *Pleasure—A Creative Approach to Life;* and Keleman, *Your Body Speaks Its Mind* and *The Human Ground.*
2. Lowen, *The Language of the Body,* p. 15.

3. Excerpted from the Esalen catalogue, spring, 1976.

4. For more material on the "open encounter process," please refer to Schutz, *Joy—Expanding Human Awareness, Here Comes Everybody,* and *Elements of Encounter.*

5. Both Schutz and Prestera have developed therapeutic systems drawn from these early experiments with the body and emotional release. See Schutz and Turner, *Evy;* and Prestera and Kurtz, *The Body Reveals.*

6. Rolf, "Structural Integration," *Systematics* 1, no. 1 (June 1963), pp. 9, 10.

7. For descriptions of the Rolfing process and theory, please refer to Rolf, *Structural Integration;* Schutz, *Here Comes Everybody;* Adam Smith, *Powers of Mind;* Prestera and Kurtz, *The Body Reveals;* and Keen, "My New Carnality."

8. In this book, I have chosen to explore and discuss the various bodymind parts and regions by ascending upward through the bodymind. This type of structure allows the development of a great many of the points that I wish to make. By utilizing this form of presentation, however, I do not wish to imply that the most appropriate order to use when working therapeutically is to begin with the feet and work upward through the bodymind. Rather, when I work with an individual I might begin my therapeutic focus at any point in the bodymind. Once begun, the order in which the therapeutic process develops is always dictated by the unique needs and characteristics of the patient. To date, I have not developed any uniform approach to this process.

CHAPTER 2. OVERVIEW

1. The possibility that personal growth can be approached as an adventure or exploration instead of a task to be achieved has been nicely discussed in the following books: Trungpa, *Cutting Through Spiritual Materialism;* Kramer, *The Passionate Mind;* Casteneda, *Tales of Power;* DeRopp, *The Master Game;* Maslow, *Toward a Psychology of Being;* Daumal, *Mount Analogue;* Shah, *Caravan of Dreams;* and Watts, *The Joyous Cosmology.*

2. Schutz, *Elements of Encounter,* pp. 23, 24.

3. I believe that we ingest and process three general types of fuel within our bodyminds. The first level on which we eat is the level of material substance. What we eat, how we eat it, and how our bodyminds are able to process it will surely affect our state of being. The second and more important level on which we fuel ourselves is the level of information. What information we ingest, how we ingest it, and how we process it will also affect our state of being. The third level on which we provide nutrition for our bodyminds is the level of energy, emotions, and spirit. This level, which I believe to be the most important, is that in which we ingest the feelings and attitudes that we need to keep ourselves feeling

healthy and happy. How we ingest them and how we are able to integrate them into our bodyminds will greatly influence our state of being.

4. For a fascinating discussion of the relationships between consciousness and environment, see Soleri, *The Bridge Between Matter and Spirit Is Matter Becoming Spirit.*

5. For more information regarding the ways in which the mind and body effect each other, refer to the following books: Wilhelm Reich, *Character Analysis;* Keleman, *Your Body Speaks Its Mind;* Prestera and Kurtz, *The Body Reveals;* Lowen, *Bioenergetics;* Barbara Brown, *New Mind, New Body—Bio-Feedback;* and Lewis and Lewis, *Psychosomatics.*

6. Enlightening discussions of the relationships between Eastern and Western approaches to the bodymind can be found in the following books: Watts, *Psychotherapy East and West;* Pelletier and Garfield, *Consciousness East and West;* Campbell, *Myths to Live By;* DeRopp, *The Master Game;* Mishlove, *The Roots of Consciousness;* White, *The Highest State of Consciousness;* and Huxley, *Island.*

7. If you are interested in doing a more in-depth psychosomatic map for yourself, refer to the interesting techniques proposed by Samuels and Bennett, *The Well Body Book.*

8. Ornstein, *The Psychology of Consciousness,* p. 52.

9. While words like "masculine" and "feminine" are entirely relative and arbitrary, they do serve some communication purposes insofar as we associate certain qualities with them. Please be aware that I am trying to steer clear of value judgments about these qualities such as "the masculine side is better or worse," or "the left side is more worthwhile or less worthwhile." Rather, I hope to show that the complementary forces of our lives, such as masculine/feminine, right/left, inner/outer, are equally beautiful and powerful in their own ways.

10. Schutz, *Here Comes Everybody,* p. 79.

11. Rapoport, "Leboyer Follow-up," pp. 14, 15.

12. Leboyer, *Birth Without Violence* and *Loving Hands.*

13. Lowen, *The Language of the Body,* p. 98.

14. An in-depth discussion of the relationships between stress and dis-ease can be found in Selye, *The Stress of Life* and *Stress Without Distress.*

15. For interesting discussions of the ways in which personal negativity can be transformed, see Trungpa, *Cutting Through Spiritual Materialism,* and Roberts, *The Nature of Personal Reality.*

16. An in-depth view of some of the clinical applications of bio-feedback can be found in Barbara Brown, *New Mind, New Body—Bio-Feedback.*

17. If you are interested in reading more about these major bodymind splits, refer to the following books: Fast, *Body Language;* Lowen, *Bioenergetics* and *The Language of the Body;* Schutz, *Here Comes Everybody;* Prestera and Kurtz, *The Body Reveals;* Keleman, *Your Body Speaks Its Mind;* Baker, *Man in the Trap;* and Ornstein, *The Psychology of Consciousness.*

CHAPTER 3. FEET AND LEGS

1. Huang, *Embrace Tiger, Return to Mountain,* p. 19.

2. For more information regarding T'ai Chi, refer to Feng and Kirk, *T'ai Chi—A Way of Centering and I Ching;* Huang, *Embrace Tiger, Return to Mountain;* and Delza, *T'ai Chi Ch'uan.*

3. Probably the best discussions of the psychological nature of grounding can be found in Keleman, *The Human Ground* and *Your Body Speaks Its Mind.*

4. Schutz, *Here Comes Everybody,* p. 77.

5. Additional material on the role that the feet play in the grounding process can be found in Lowen, *The Language of the Body;* Baker, *Man in the Trap;* and Prestera and Kurtz, *The Body Reveals.*

6. Schutz, *Here Comes Everybody,* pp. 77, 78.

7. Lowen, *The Language of the Body,* p. 101.

8. Detailed discussions of foot reflexology and its clinical applications can be found in Ingham, *Stories the Feet Can Tell* and *Stories the Feet Have Told;* and Carter, *Helping Yourself with Foot Reflexology.*

9. For more information regarding zone therapy and "chi" energy, see De Langre, *The First Book of Do-In,* and Mann, *Acupuncture—Cure of Many Diseases.*

10. The relationship between stress and dis-ease is well presented in Selye, *The Stress of Life* and *Stress Without Distress.*

11. The books on yoga that I have found to be most helpful are Hittleman, *Introduction to Yoga,* as a simple beginner's yoga manual; Vishnudevananda, *The Complete Illustrated Book of Yoga,* and Satchidananda, *Integral Yoga Hatha,* for their well-illustrated, easy-to-follow texts and lessons; Marga, *Teaching Asanas,* for its holistic and well-rounded approach to yoga; Iyengar, *Light on Yoga,* for its innovative approach to yoga and its comprehensive sections of prescriptive postures; Mishra, *Fundamentals of Yoga* and *Yoga Sutras,* for their enlightening discussions of yoga theory and psychology; Kramer, *The Passionate Mind,* for its clear and provocative presentation of contemporary yoga philosophy; and Rama, Ballentine, and Ayaja, *Yoga and Psychotherapy,* for its masterful presentation of some of the ways that yoga can be utilized in psychotherapy.

12. For more in-depth discussions of Eastern/Western approaches to growth, see Watts, *Psychotherapy East and West;* Trungpa, *Cutting Through Spiritual Materialism;* Mishlove, *The Roots of Consciousness;* Campbell, *Myths to Live By;* DeRopp, *The Master Game;* Naranjo, *The One Quest;* Kramer, *The Passionate Mind;* Metzner, *Maps of Consciousness;* and Rama, Ballentine, and Ayaja, *Yoga and Psychotherapy.*

13. See Samuels and Bennett, *The Well Body Book,* for a simple and worthwhile approach to seeing the body as a self-healing machine.

14. For additional material on the psychosomatic nature of the legs,

see Baker, *Man in the Trap;* Lowen, *The Language of the Body* and *Bioenerget-ics;* Prestera and Kurtz, *The Body Reveals;* and Schutz, *Here Comes Every-body.*

CHAPTER 4. PELVIS

1. Rolf, *Structural Integration.*
2. Lowen, *Bioenergetics* and *The Language of the Body.*
3. For additional information on tantra, Kundalini energy, and the Kundalini chakras, see Garrison, *Tantra: The Yoga of Sex;* Rama, Ballentine, and Ajaya, *Yoga and Psychotherapy;* Rawson, *Tantra;* Haich, *Sexual Energy and Yoga;* Leadbeater, *The Chakras;* Krishna, *Kundalini;* Rendel, *Introduction to the Chakras;* Campbell, *Myths to Live By* and "Seven Levels of Consciousness"; Schutz, *Here Comes Everybody;* Mishlove, *The Roots of Consciousness;* Rosenberg, *Total Orgasm;* and William Thompson, *Passages About Earth.*
4. It is not within the scope of this book to elaborate more fully on the ways in which each of the chakras corresponds to sound, color, vibration, etc. For explorations of these relationships, see Leadbeater, *The Chakras;* Rendel, *Introduction to the Chakras;* Garrison, *Tantra: The Yoga of Sex;* Rama, Ballentine, and Ajaya, *Yoga and Psychotherapy;* and Campbell, *Myths to Live By.*
5. Schutz, *Here Comes Everybody,* p. 65.
6. Baker, *Man in the Trap,* pp. 41, 42.
7. For additional information on holding in the anal region, see Baker, *Man in the Trap;* Lowen, *Bioenergetics, Pleasure—A Creative Approach to Life, The Language of the Body,* and *The Betrayal of the Body;* Prestera and Kurtz, *The Body Reveals;* and Schutz, *Here Comes Everybody.*
8. Wilhelm Reich, *The Function of the Orgasm,* p. 4.
9. Wilhelm Reich, "Die Therapeutische Bedentung der Genital Li-bido," *International Journal of Psycho-analysis,* 10 (1924), translated by Boadella in *Wilhelm Reich: The Evolution of His Work,* p. 16.
10. Walt Anderson, "Strange Prophet," pp. 24–29.
11. Rosenberg, *Total Orgasm,* pp. 30–34.
12. See Laughingbird, "SAGE."
13. For more information on the SAGE Project, write to The Sage Project, Claremont Office Park, 41 Tunnel Road, Berkeley, California 94705.
14. Boadella, *Wilhelm Reich: The Evolution of His Work,* p. 30.
15. The following are those of Wilhelm Reich's books which I have found most illuminating: *The Cancer Biopathy, Character Analysis, The Murder of Christ, Selected Writings: An Introduction to Orgonomy, Sex-Pol: Essays 1929–1934, The Sexual Revolution, Cosmic Superimposition, The Discovery of the Orgone, Ether, God and Devil/Cosmic Superimposition, The Function of the Orgasm,* and *Listen, Little Man.* In addition, there have been a great many

books written about Reich's life and work. I feel that the best of these are Boadella, *Wilhelm Reich: The Evolution of His Work;* Baker, *Man in the Trap;* Cattier, *The Life and Work of Wilhelm Reich;* and Raknes, *Wilhelm Reich and Orgonomy.*

16. William Thompson, *Passages About Earth,* p. 107.

17. Garrison, *Tantra: The Yoga of Sex,* p. 114.

18. Actually, I have discovered some disagreement as to whether the tantric lovers experience orgasm or not. Some sources say that both lovers simultaneously experience a spontaneous orgasm after a specific amount of time has elapsed. Other sources say that although the lovers do experience an energetic climax or zenith, it is *not* actually an orgasm that they are feeling.

19. William Thompson, *Passages About Earth,* p. 109.

20. For additional information on the tantric approach to sexuality, see Garrison, *Tantra: The Yoga of Sex;* William Thompson, *Passages About Earth;* Haich, *Sexual Energy and Yoga;* Campbell, *Myths to Live By;* Rama, Ballentine, and Ajaya, *Yoga and Psychotherapy;* Rosenberg, *Total Orgasm;* and Huxley, *Island.*

21. There are several books that offer experiential exercises that I have found to be extremely helpful in freeing myself up. They are Rosenberg, *Total Orgasm;* Rush, *Getting Clear: Body Work for Women;* Geba, *Breathe Away Your Tension;* Gunther, *Sense Relaxation Below Your Mind* and *What to Do Till the Messiah Comes;* and Marga, *Teaching Asanas.*

CHAPTER 5. ABDOMINAL REGION AND LOWER BACK

1. For descriptions of the various Reichian and bioenergetic segments, see Wilhelm Reich, *Character Analysis;* Baker, *Man in the Trap;* and Lowen, *Bioenergetics* and *The Language of the Body.*

2. For more detailed information on this Kundalini chakra, refer to Leadbeater, *The Chakras;* Rendel, *Introduction to the Chakras;* Rama, Ballentine, and Ajaya, *Yoga and Psychotherapy;* Schutz, *Here Comes Everybody;* Campbell, *Myths To Live By;* and Garrison, *Tantra: The Yoga of Sex.*

3. In a way, the characteristics of the first three chakras can be compared with the organizing principles of three popular Western psychological schools: behavioristic, Freudian, and Adlerian. The first chakra, with its emphasis on the give-and-take material aspects of human existence, parallels the theory and technique of the behavioristic school as epitomized in the work of B. F. Skinner. The second chakra, with its sexual and interpersonal focus, corresponds to the Freudian or Reichian line of thought. And the third chakra, which is focused on feelings, sexual behavior, and power, can be compared with the Adlerian school of psychology. Campbell elaborates more fully on this point in *Myths to Live By.*

4. Campbell, *Myths to Live By,* p. 111.

5. This emotional energy cycle has been well explained by William Schutz in *Elements of Encounter.*

6. For an enlightening discussion of the possible relationships between tension and disease, see Selye, *The Stress of Life* and *Stress Without Distress.*

7. Schutz, *Here Comes Everybody,* p. 81.

8. While there have been numerous reported cases of the spontaneous release of emotion during a Rolfing treatment, most Rolfers are not trained or inclined to work with the emotional material as it comes up. William Schutz has developed a method whereby Rolfing is combined with guided-imagery techniques to provide a situation in which stored feelings can both be released and worked through. See Schutz and Turner, *Evy.*

9. While regurgitating is something that many of us consider unpleasant and unhealthy, there are bodymind approaches that recognize its cleansing value. For example, in certain phases of bioenergetic therapy, the patient is encouraged to induce himself to regurgitate as a way of releasing tension and eliminating blocked energy. Similarly, there are yogic cleansing exercises called "kriyas" that are designed specifically for regurgitative elimination.

10. For additional information about Rolfing, see Rolf, *Structural Integration;* Schutz, *Here Comes Everybody;* Adam Smith, *Powers of Mind;* and Keen, "My New Carnality."

11. For a discussion of the way to deal with blocked anger in the encounter-group setting, see Schutz, *Joy—Expanding Human Awareness, Here Comes Everybody,* and *Elements of Encounter;* and Rogers, *On Encounter Groups.*

12. See also Roberts, *The Seth Material* and *Seth Speaks—The Eternal Validity of the Soul.*

13. Roberts, *The Nature of Personal Reality,* pp. 160–62.

14. In my own experience with yoga and T'ai Chi, I have discovered that certain movements, positions, and postures (asanas) work directly on specific bodymind parts. As a result, when I utilize these techniques with myself or with my patients, I try to prescribe the correct exercise or exercises for the unique needs of the person.

15. For detailed descriptions of some of these exercises, see Lowen, *Bioenergetics* and *The Betrayal of the Body;* Keleman, *Your Body Speaks Its Mind;* Baker, *Man in the Trap;* Janov, *The Primal Scream;* and Schutz, *Joy —Expanding Human Awareness.*

16. Lowen, *Bioenergetics,* p. 234.

17. For information and exercises on relieving lower-back pain refer to Lowen, *Bioenergetics;* Schutz, *Here Comes Everybody;* Marga, *Teaching Asanas;* Iyengar, *Light on Yoga;* Vishnudevananda, *The Complete Illustrated Book of Yoga;* Rama, Ballentine, and Ajaya, *Yoga and Psychotherapy;* Sharma, *Yoga for Backaches;* Rush, *Getting Clear: Body Work for Women;*

Rosenberg, *Total Orgasm;* Hearn, *You Are as Young as Your Spine;* Shuman and Staab, *Your Aching Back;* Enelow, *The Joy of Physical Freedom;* Dintenfass, *Chiropractic—A Modern Way to Health;* and Prestera and Kurtz, *The Body Reveals.*

18. Since yoga is the bodymind method with which I am most fluent, I frequently use the yoga postures in my diagnosis procedure. When I have ascertained which muscles are tight or unconscious, I then proceed to work toward bodymind balance and vitality in a holistic fashion. I might or might not use yoga asanas for the therapeutic work.

19. Wilhelm Reich, *Character Analysis,* p. 381.

20. Baker, *Man in the Trap,* p. 88.

21. For additional information on the diaphragm region of the bodymind, see Wilhelm Reich, *Character Analysis;* Baker, *Man in the Trap;* and Lowen, *Bioenergetics, The Language of the Body* and *The Betrayal of the Body.*

22. Schutz, *Here Comes Everybody,* p. 194.

23. See Geba, *Breathe Away Your Tension,* for practical breathing exercises and techniques.

CHAPTER 6. CHEST CAVITY

1. See Wilhelm Reich, *Character Analysis.*

2. Information and exercises on pranayama can be found in Garrison, *Tantra: The Yoga of Sex;* Vishnudevananda, *The Complete Illustrated Book of Yoga;* Mishra, *Fundamentals of Yoga;* and Geba, *Breathe Away Your Tension.*

3. Perls, Hefferline, and Goodman, *Gestalt Therapy,* pp. 128, 130.

4. For more information on this documentary or any other SAGE material, please write to The SAGE Project, Claremont Office Park, 41 Tunnel Road, Berkeley, California 94705.

5. For a more in-depth discussion of the Anahata chakra, refer to Rama, Ballentine, and Ajaya, *Yoga and Psychotherapy;* Garrison, *Tantra: The Yoga of Sex;* Leadbeater, *The Chakras;* Rendel, *Introduction to the Chakras;* Campbell, *Myths to Live By;* and William Thompson, *Passages About Earth.*

6. I frequently fast for several days at a time to cleanse my body of accumulated toxins. During the fast, I often find that I am more relaxed and introspective than usual. In addition, the abstention from eating always encourages me to pay close attention to my body. Enlightening discussions of the fasting process can be found in Airola, *Are You Confused?;* Bragg, *The Miracle of Fasting;* and Jensen, *The Science and Practice of Iridology.*

7. An interesting discussion of the psychosomatic aspects of love and faith can be found in Lowen, *Depression and the Body.*

8. For a fascinating collection of essays on love, see Otto, ed., *Love Today.*

9. Lowen, *The Language of the Body,* p. 102.

10. See Baker, *Man in the Trap.*

11. For additional information on the psychosomatic nature of the chest, refer to Prestera and Kurtz, *The Body Reveals;* Lowen, *The Language of the Body;* Baker, *Man in the Trap;* Schutz, *Here Comes Everybody;* and Keleman, *Your Body Speaks Its Mind.*

CHAPTER 7. SHOULDERS AND ARMS

1. Boadella, *Wilhelm Reich: The Evolution of His Work,* p. 42.
2. See Lewis and Lewis, *Psychosomatics.*
3. For additional information on the psychosomatic nature of the shoulders, see Prestera and Kurtz, *The Body Reveals;* Lowen, *The Language of the Body;* and Alexander, *The Resurrection of the Body.*
4. Keen, "A Conversation About Ego Destruction with Oscar Ichazo," *Psychology Today,* July 1973, p. 68.
5. Wilhelm Reich, *Character Analysis,* p. 378.
6. Additional material on the arms and hands can be found in Prestera and Kurtz, *The Body Reveals;* Lowen, *Bioenergetics* and *The Language of the Body;* and Keleman, *Your Body Speaks Its Mind.*
7. While palmistry is not an area about which I know a great deal, I have been impressed with some of the ways the hands can be used in diagnosing the entire bodymind. For more information on this subject, see Broekman, *The Complete Encyclopedia of Practical Palmistry;* Wolff, *The Hand in Psychological Diagnosis;* and Ellis, *The Doctor Who Looked at Hands.*
8. Rodale and Staff, *Encyclopedia of Common Diseases,* p. 169.
9. A nice discussion of personal space can be found in Fast, *Body Language.*
10. Gestalt therapy is heavily indebted to the work of Wilhelm Reich for the way in which it places a great deal of emphasis on nonverbal behavior. The Gestalt emphases on self-responsibility, bodymind unity, and growth through integration have become crucial components of my own life and work. For more information on Gestalt therapy, see Perls, *Ego, Hunger and Aggression* and *In and Out the Garbage Pail;* and Perls, Hefferline, and Goodman, *Gestalt Therapy.*
11. Fast, *Body Language,* pp. 14–16.
12. See Dintenfass, *Chiropractic—A Modern Way to Health.*
13. For additional information on the psychosomatic nature of the upper back, refer to Lowen, *Bioenergetics* and *The Language of the Body;* Baker, *Man in the Trap;* Prestera and Kurtz, *The Body Reveals;* Keleman, *Your Body Speaks Its Mind;* Shuman and Staab, *Your Aching Back;* Hearn, *You Are as Young as Your Spine;* Iyengar, *Light on Yoga;* Marga, *Teaching Asanas;* and Sharma, *Yoga for Backaches.*

CHAPTER 8. NECK, THROAT, AND JAW

1. "Spiritual," as it is used here, is not meant to refer to any particular institution or religious doctrine. Rather, I use the word to refer to the

feelings of connectedness and oneness that I feel when I have transcended my usual tensions and distractions and have entered into a state of calm, clarity, and peace. In this way, spirituality can be viewed as a state of being or a state of awareness rather than a prescribed set of laws or forms. For more in-depth discussions on this topic, refer to Maslow, *Religions, Values, and Peak-Experiences;* James, *The Varieties of Religious Experience;* Campbell, *Myths to Live By;* Trungpa, *Cutting Through Spiritual Materialism;* Watts, *The Joyous Cosmology;* Roberts, *Seth Speaks—The Eternal Validity of the Soul;* DeRopp, *The Master Game;* and Dass, *Be Here Now.*

2. For more information on the fifth chakra, "Vishuddha," refer to Rama, Ballentine, and Ajaya, *Yoga and Psychotherapy;* Leadbeater, *The Chakras;* Rendel, *Introduction to the Chakras;* Campbell, *Myths to Live By;* William Thompson, *Passages About Earth;* Schutz, *Here Comes Everybody;* Garrison, *Tantra: The Yoga of Sex;* and Krishna, *Kundalini, Evolutionary Energy in Man.*

3. Lowen, *The Language of the Body*, p. 105.

4. *Ibid.*

5. For additional information on the psychosomatic qualities of the neck, see Lowen, *Bioenergetics* and *The Language of the Body;* Prestera and Kurtz, *The Body Reveals;* Schutz, *Here Comes Everybody;* Baker, *Man in the Trap;* and Rolf, *Structural Integration.*

6. Schutz, *Here Comes Everybody,* pp. 85, 86.

7. Normally the jaw is Rolfed during the seventh treatment hour. Actually it was quite unorthodox for Prestera to do what he did in this situation.

8. For an in-depth discussion of the ways psychodrama can be used therapeutically, refer to Greenberg, *Psychodrama Theory and Therapy;* Moreno, *Who Shall Survive?;* and Schutz, *Elements of Encounter.*

9. It is interesting to note that F. M. Alexander, the creator of the Alexander technique, was himself a stutterer. He discusses this problem in detail in *The Resurrection of the Body.*

10. For additional information on the psychosomatic nature of the jaw, see Prestera and Kurtz, *The Body Reveals;* Baker, *Man in the Trap;* Lowen, *Bioenergetics* and *The Language of the Body;* Schutz, *Here Comes Everybody;* Mar, *Face Reading;* and Alexander, *The Resurrection of the Body.*

11. See Feldenkrais, *Awareness Through Movement* and *Body and Mature Behavior.*

12. See Feldenkrais, *Awareness Through Movement,* and Schutz, *Elements of Encounter,* for examples of these exercises.

13. Schutz, *Elements of Encounter,* pp. 27, 28.

14. The Feldenkrais exercises are remarkably similar to yoga asanas in that their primary purpose is self-awareness through self-exploration, not self-control through self-punishment.

15. Some of the most provocative discussions of the ways self-image influences behavior can be found in Castaneda's books: *Journey to Ixtlan, A Separate Reality, Tales of Power,* and *The Teachings of Don Juan;* Roberts,

The Nature of Personal Reality, The Seth Material, and *Seth Speaks—The Eternal Validity of the Soul;* Campbell, *Myths to Live By;* Pearce, *The Crack in the Cosmic Egg;* Abbott, *Flatland: A Romance of Many Dimensions;* Huxley, *The Doors of Perception* and *Heaven and Hell;* May, *Man's Search for Himself;* Trungpa, *Meditation in Action;* and Lilly, *Programming and Metaprogramming in the Human Biocomputer* and *The Center of the Cyclone.*

CHAPTER 9. FACE AND HEAD

1. One of the problems with breaking the bodymind up into segments, as I have done, is that the face becomes divided into two chapters. For now, please remember that the face is made up of the oral and ocular segments.
2. Lowen, *Bioenergetics,* pp. 89, 90.
3. For additional information on the way in which emotional trauma blocks full bodymind awareness, see Wilhelm Reich, *Character Analysis;* Baker, *Man in the Trap;* Boadella, *Wilhelm Reich: The Evolution of His Work;* Lowen, *Bioenergetics, The Language of the Body, The Betrayal of the Body, Pleasure—A Creative Approach to Life, Depression and the Body,* and *Love and Orgasm;* Prestera and Kurtz, *The Body Reveals;* Keleman, *Your Body Speaks Its Mind* and *The Human Ground;* Rama, Ballentine, and Ajaya, *Yoga and Psychotherapy;* Schutz, *Here Comes Everybody* and *Joy—Expanding Human Awareness;* Janov, *The Primal Scream;* and Fast, *Body Language.*
4. See Mar, *Face Reading.*
5. Baker, *Man in the Trap,* p. 76.
6. See Bates, *The Bates Method for Better Eyesight Without Glasses;* C. Kelly, *New Techniques of Vision Improvement;* Jackson, *Seeing Yourself See;* and Lowen, *Bioenergetics.*
7. For additional information on the psychosomatic nature of the eyes, refer to Kelly, *New Techniques of Vision Improvement;* Bates, *The Bates Method for Better Eyesight Without Glasses;* Jackson, *Seeing Yourself See;* Baker, *Man in the Trap;* Lowen, *The Language of the Body* and *Bioenergetics;* Prestera and Kurtz, *The Body Reveals;* and Janov, *The Primal Scream.*
8. Jensen, *The Science and Practice of Iridology,* p. 1.
9. For more information on the use of the eye in bodymind diagnosis, see Jensen, *The Science and Practice of Iridology.*
10. Lowen, *Bioenergetics,* p. 90.
11. For additional information on the psychosomatic nature of the forehead, see Lowen, *The Language of the Body* and *Bioenergetics;* Prestera and Kurtz, *The Body Reveals;* Baker, *Man in the Trap;* and Schutz, *Here Comes Everybody.*
12. For a more detailed discussion of the various qualities of the sixth chakra, "Ajna," refer to Krishna, *Kundalini, Evolutionary Energy in Man;* Rendel, *Introduction to the Chakras;* Leadbeater, *The Chakras;* Rama, Ballentine, and Ajaya, *Yoga and Psychotherapy;* Garrison, *Tantra: The Yoga of Sex;* Campbell, *Myths to Live By;* William Thompson, *Passages About Earth;* and Mishlove, *The Roots of Consciousness.*

13. While it is not within the scope of this book to present an in-depth analysis of this point, I would like to mention that there has been some fascinating research and speculation on the various alternative modes of perceiving. In addition, there is a wealth of information that points to numerous ways in which the brain and nervous system might relate holistically to the rest of the bodymind. For additional information on these topics, refer to: Barbara Brown, *New Mind, New Body—Bio-Feedback;* DeRopp, *The Master Game;* Feldenkrais, *Awareness Through Movement;* Lilly, *The Center of the Cyclone* and *Simulations of God;* Mishlove, *The Roots of Consciousness;* Naranjo, *The One Quest;* Samuels and Samuels, *Seeing with the Mind's Eye;* Adam Smith, *Powers of Mind;* Tart, ed., *Altered States of Consciousness;* White, *The Highest State of Consciousness;* Anderson and Savary, *Passages: A Guide for Pilgrims of the Mind;* Campbell, *Myths to Live By;* Castaneda, *Journey to Ixtlan, A Separate Reality, Tales of Power,* and *The Teachings of Don Juan;* Hunter, *The Storming of the Mind;* Huxley, *The Doors of Perception* and *Heaven and Hell;* Jonas, *Visceral Learning;* Jung, *On the Nature of the Psyche* and *Synchronicity: An Acausal Connecting Principle;* Koestler, *The Roots of Coincidence;* LeShan, *How to Meditate;* Masters and Houston, *Mind Games: The Guide to Inner Space* and *The Varieties of Psychedelic Experience;* Muses and Young, *Consciousness and Reality;* Pearce, *The Crack in the Cosmic Egg;* Roberts, *The Nature of Personal Reality, The Seth Material,* and *Seth Speaks—The Eternal Validity of the Soul;* Sivananda, *Gyana Yoga;* Tompkins and Bird, *The Secret Life of Plants;* Weil, *The Natural Mind;* Neumann, *The Origins and History of Consciousness;* Ornstein, *The Nature of Human Consciousness* and *The Psychology of Consciousness;* Pelletier and Garfield, *Consciousness East and West.*

14. For additional information on the psychic senses, refer to Castaneda, *Journey to Ixtlan, A Separate Reality, Tales of Power,* and *The Teachings of Don Juan;* Huxley, *The Doors of Perception* and *Heaven and Hell;* Krishna, *Kundalini, Evolutionary Energy in Man;* Pearce, *The Crack in the Cosmic Egg;* Gibson and Bigson, *The Complete Illustrated Book of the Psychic Sciences;* Hansel, *E.S.P.: A Scientific Evaluation;* Jung, *Synchronicity;* Koestler, *The Roots of Coincidence;* LeShan, *How to Meditate;* Mishlove, *The Roots of Consciousness;* Moss, *The Probability of the Impossible;* Ornstein, *The Nature of Human Consciousness* and *The Psychology of Consciousness;* Ostrander and Schroeder, *Psychic Discoveries Behind the Iron Curtain;* Porter, *Psychic Development;* Puharich, *Beyond Telepathy* and *Uri;* Rhine, *New World of the Mind* and *The Reach of the Mind;* Adam Smith, *Powers of Mind;* Sinclair, *Mental Radio;* Tart, ed., *Altered States of Consciousness;* Tompkins and Bird, *The Secret Life of Plants;* White, *The Highest State of Consciousness;* and Wilson, *The Mind Parasites.*

15. Huxley, *The Doors of Perception* and *Heaven and Hell,* pp. 22–23.

16. See Adam Smith, *Powers of Mind.*

17. Of all the books on meditation, the two that I like best are LeShan, *How to Meditate;* and Trungpa, *Meditation in Action.*

18. Kramer, *The Passionate Mind,* p. 101.

19. See Maslow, *Toward a Psychology of Being* and *Religions, Values, and Peak-Experiences.*
20. See Adam Smith, *Powers of Mind;* Trungpa, *Cutting Through Spiritual Materialism;* and Kramer, *The Passionate Mind.*

CHAPTER 10. BODYMIND

1. While it has not been appropriate to present descriptions of the other glands of the body, they are, in descending order: the pituitary gland, the thyroid and parathyroid glands, the thymus gland, the adrenal glands, the pancreas, and the gonads. For relevant and simple discussions of these glands, see Ananda Marga, *Teaching Asanas,* pp. 47–50.
2. *Ibid.*, p. 47.
3. For additional information on the seventh chakra, "Sahasrara," refer to Rama, Ballentine, and Ajaya, *Yoga and Psychotherapy;* Krishna, *Kundalini, Evolutionary Energy in Man;* Leadbeater, *The Chakras;* Rendel, *Introduction to the Chakras;* Campbell, *Myths to Live By;* Garrison, *Tantra: The Yoga of Sex;* Thompson, *Passages About Earth;* and Schutz, *Here Comes Everybody.*
4. Campbell, "Seven Levels of Consciousness," pp. 76–78.
5. *Ibid.*, pp. 3, 4.
6. *Ibid.*, p. 1.
7. *Ibid.*
8. *Ibid.*, p. 3.
9. The belief that humankind is entering into a period of evolutionary transformation has been expressed by an extensive collection of great thinkers and visionaries. Discussions of this perspective can be found in the following books: Arguelles, *The Transformative Vision;* Aurobindo, *The Future Evolution of Man;* Teilhard de Chardin, *Building the Earth;* Teilhard de Chardin, *The Phenomenon of Man;* DeRopp, *The Master Game;* Fuller, *Utopia or Oblivion;* Hunter, *The Storming of the Mind;* Koestler, *The Roots of Coincidence;* Krishna, *Kundalini, Evolutionary Energy in Man;* Kuhn, *The Structure of Scientific Revolutions;* Leonard, *The Transformation;* Murphy, *Human Potentialities;* Muses and Young, *Consciousness and Reality;* Naranjo, *The One Quest;* Ouspensky, *The Psychology of Man's Possible Evolution;* Pearce, *The Crack in the Cosmic Egg;* Charles Reich, *The Greening of America;* Spangler, *Revelation;* Steiner, *Knowledge of the Higher Worlds and Its Attainment;* William Thompson, *At the Edge of History* and *Passages About Earth;* Trungpa and Guenther, *The Dawn of Tantra;* and White, *The Highest State of Consciousness.*
10. I have discovered that the most fascinating speculations on the human evolutionary process are to be found in contemporary science fiction books. For examples, refer to Clarke, *Childhood's End;* Wilson, *The Mind Parasites;* Stapleton, *Last and First Men* and *Star Maker;* Silverbert, *Son of Man;* Heinlein, *Stranger in a Strange Land;* Herbert, *Dune;* Asimov, *Foundation, Foundation and Empire,* and *Second Foundation;* and Abbott, *Flatland.*

11. The living human organism does not ever exist as a static structure. For it to do so, all internal and external life and motion would have to cease and the persistent flow of time would have to freeze. Since neither of these possibilities is very likely, human structure becomes an abstract concept that we have created with our thoughts and cameras in an attempt to isolate and capture time, thereby separating ourselves from the continually pulsating flow of life within which we are immersed. In essence, structure can be seen as frozen function.

12. See Ram Dass, *The Only Dance There Is.*

BIBLIOGRAPHY

Abbott, Edwin. *Flatland: A Romance of Many Dimensions.* New York: Dover Publications, 1952.

Alexander, F. M. *The Resurrection of the Body.* New York: Dell Publishing Co., 1971.

Anderson, Marianne, and Savary, Louis. *Passages: A Guide for Pilgrims of the Mind.* New York: Harper & Row, 1973.

Anderson, Walt. "Strange Prophet." *Human Behavior,* January 1976, pp. 24–29.

Arguelles, José. *The Transformative Vision: Reflections on the Nature and History of Human Expression.* Berkeley: Shambala Publications, 1975.

Asimov, Isaac. *Foundation.* New York: Avon Books, 1966.

————. *Foundation and Empire.* New York: Avon Books, 1966.

————. *Second Foundation.* New York: Avon Books, 1966.

Assagioli, Roberto. *Psychosynthesis.* New York: Viking Press, 1971.

Aurobindo, Sri. *The Future Evolution of Man: The Divine Life upon Earth.* Wheaton, Ill.: Theosophical Publishing House, 1974.

Baker, Elsworth. *Man in the Trap: The Causes of Blocked Sexual Energy.* New York: Avon Books, 1974.

Bates, W. H. *The Bates Method for Better Eyesight Without Glasses.* New York: Pyramid Books, 1971.

Bateson, Gregory. *Steps to an Ecology of Mind.* New York: Ballantine Books, 1972.

Behanan, Kovoor. *Yoga, A Scientific Evaluation.* New York: Dover Publications, 1964.

Birdwhistell, Ray. *Kinesics and Context: Essays on Body Motion Communication.*
Philadelphia: University of Pennsylvania Press, 1970.
Bleibtreu, John. *The Parable of the Beast.* New York: Collier Books, 1971.
Blofeld, John. *The Tantric Mysticism of Tibet.* New York: E. P. Dutton &
Co., 1970.
────. *The Zen Teaching of Huang Po.* New York: Grove Press, 1958.
Boadella, David. *Wilhelm Reich: The Evolution of His Work.* Chicago: Henry
Regnery Co., 1974.
Boyd, Doug. *Swami.* New York: Random House, 1976.
Bragg, Paul. *The Miracle of Fasting.* Desert Hot Springs, Cal.: Health
Science, 1976.
Broekman, Marcel. *The Complete Encyclopedia of Practical Palmistry.* Engle-
wood Cliffs, N.J.: Prentice-Hall, 1972.
Brooks, Charles. *Sensory Awareness: The Rediscovery of Experiencing.* New
York: Viking Press, 1974.
Brown, Barbara. *New Mind, New Body—Bio-Feedback: New Directions for the
Mind.* New York: Harper & Row, 1974.
Brown, George. *Human Teaching for Human Learning: An Introduction to
Confluent Education.* New York: Viking Press, 1973.
Brown, Norman, *Love's Body.* New York: Vintage Books, 1968.
Bucke, Richard. *Cosmic Consciousness.* New York: E. P. Dutton & Co.,
1969.
Burr, Harold. *The Fields of Life: Our Links with the Universe.* New York:
Ballantine Books, 1973.
Campbell, Joseph. *The Hero with a Thousand Faces.* 2d ed. Princeton, N.J.:
Princeton University Press, 1968.
────. *Myths to Live By.* New York: Bantam Books, 1973.
────. "Seven Levels of Consciousness." *Psychology Today,* December
1975, pp. 76–78.
Carter, Mildred. *Helping Yourself with Foot Reflexology.* West Nyack, N.Y.:
Parker Publishing Co., 1969.
Castaneda, Carlos. *Journey to Ixtlan: The Lessons of Don Juan.* New York:
Simon & Schuster, 1973.
────. *A Separate Reality: Further Conversations with Don Juan.* New York:
Simon & Schuster, 1971.
────. *Tales of Power.* New York: Simon & Schuster, 1974.
────. *The Teachings of Don Juan: A Yaqui Way of Knowledge.* New York:
Ballantine Books, 1974.
Cattier, Michel. *The Life and Work of Wilhelm Reich.* New York: Avon
Books, 1973.
Cayce, Edgar. *Auras: An Essay on the Meaning of Colors.* Virginia Beach, Va.:
A.R.E. Press, 1973.
Chaitow, Leon. *Osteopathy, Head to Toe Health Through Manipulation.* Wel-
lingborough, Northamptonshire: Thorsons Publishers, 1974.
Clarke, Arthur C. *Childhood's End.* New York: Ballantine Books, 1972.
Daumal, René. *Mount Analogue.* San Francisco: City Lights Books, 1971.

Davis, Martha. *Understanding Body Movement.* New York: Arno Press, 1972.

DeLangre, Jacques. *The First Book of Do-In.* Hollywood, Cal.: Happiness Press, 1971.

———. *The Second Book of Do-In.* Hollywood, Cal.: Happiness Press, 1976.

Delza, Sophia. *T'ai Chi Ch'uan: An Ancient Chinese Way of Exercise to Achieve Health and Tranquility.* New York: Cornerstone Library, 1972.

DeRopp, Robert. *The Master Game: Pathways to Higher Consciousness Beyond the Drug Experience.* New York: Dell Publishing Co., 1968.

Dintenfass, Julius. *Chiropractic: A Modern Way to Health.* New York: Pyramid Books, 1970.

Downing, George. *The Massage Book.* New York: Random House and Berkeley: The Bookworks, 1972.

———. *Massage and Meditation.* New York: Random House and Berkeley: The Bookworks, 1974.

Durkheim, Emile. *The Elementary Forms of the Religious Life.* New York: Free Press, 1967.

Ehret, Arnold. *Rational Fasting.* New York: Benedict Lust Publications, 1971.

Eliade, Mircea. *The Sacred and the Profane: The Nature of Religion.* New York: Harper & Row, 1961.

———. *Yoga: Immortality and Freedom.* Princeton, N.J.: Princeton University Press, 1970.

Elkind, David. "Wilhelm Reich—Psychoanalyst as Revolutionary." *New York Times Magazine,* April 18, 1971, pp. 25–76.

Ellis, John. *The Doctor Who Looked at Hands.* New York: Arc Books, 1971.

Enelow, Gertrude. *The Joy of Physical Freedom.* Chicago: Henry Regnery Co., 1973.

Evans-Wentz, W. Y., ed. *The Tibetan Book of the Dead.* New York: Oxford University Press, 1974.

Fadiman, James, and Frager, Robert. *Personality and Personal Growth.* New York: Harper & Row, 1976.

Fadiman, James, and Kewman, Donald. *Exploring Madness: Experience, Theory, and Research.* Monterey, Cal.: Brooks/Cole Publishing Co., 1973.

Fast, Julius. *Body Language.* New York: M. Evans & Co., 1970.

Feldenkrais, Moshe. *Awareness Through Movement: Health Exercises for Personal Growth.* New York: Harper & Row, 1972.

———. *Body and Mature Behavior: A Study of Anxiety, Sex, Gravitation and Learning.* New York: International Universities Press, 1949.

Feng, Gia-Fu, and Kirk, Jerome. *T'ai Chi: A Way of Centering* and *I Ching.* London: Collier Books, 1970.

Fisher, Seymour. *Body Consciousness: You Are What You Feel.* Englewood Cliffs, N.J.: Prentice-Hall, 1973.

Fromm, Erich. *The Art of Loving.* New York: Bantam Books, 1967.

Fuller, R. Buckminster. *Utopia or Oblivion: The Prospects for Humanity.* New York: Bantam Books, 1969.

Furst, Jeffrey. *Edgar Cayce's Story of Attitudes and Emotions.* New York: Berkeley Publishing Corp., 1974.

Gallwey, Timothy. *The Inner Game of Tennis.* New York: Random House, 1976.

Garrison, Omar. *Tantra: The Yoga of Sex.* New York: Causeway Books, 1964.

Geba, Bruno. *Breathe Away Your Tension: An Introduction to Gestalt Body Awareness Therapy.* New York: Random House and Berkeley: The Bookworks, 1973.

Gibran, Kahlil. *The Prophet.* New York: Alfred A. Knopf, 1971.

Gibson, Walter, and Bigson, Litka. *The Complete Illustrated Book of the Psychic Sciences.* New York: Pocket Books, 1974.

Golas, Thaddeus. *The Lazy Man's Guide to Enlightenment.* Palo Alto, Cal.: Seed Center, 1973.

Green, Celia. *Out-of-the-Body Experiences.* New York: Ballantine Books, 1973.

Greenberg, Ira A. *Psychodrama Theory and Therapy.* New York: Behavioral Publications, 1974.

Grof, Stanislav. *Realms of the Human Unconscious: Observations from LSD Research.* New York: Viking Press, 1975.

Gunther, Bernard. *Sense Relaxation Below Your Mind.* New York: Collier Books, 1968.

———. *What to Do Till the Messiah Comes.* New York: Collier Books, 1971.

Gurdjieff, G. I. *Beelzebub's Tales to His Grandson, Books 1, 2, 3.* New York: E. P. Dutton & Co., 1973.

Haich, Elisabeth. *Sexual Energy and Yoga.* New York: A.S.I. Publishers, 1972.

Hall, Calvin, and Nordby, Vernon. *A Primer of Jungian Psychology.* New York: New American Library, 1973.

Hanna, Thomas. *Bodies in Revolt: A Primer in Somatic Thinking.* New York: Dell Publishing Co., 1972.

Hansel, C. E. M. *E.S.P.: A Scientific Evaluation.* New York: Charles Scribner's Sons, 1966.

Hearn, Editha. *You Are as Young as Your Spine.* New York: Gramercy Press, 1976.

Heckler, Richard. *The Mind/Body Interface.* San Francisco: Freeperson Press, 1975.

Heinlein, Robert A. *Stranger in a Strange Land.* New York: Berkeley Publishing Corp., 1969.

Herbert, Frank. *Dune.* New York: Ace Books, 1965.

Herrigel, Eugen. *Zen.* New York: McGraw-Hill Book Co., 1964.

Hesse, Herman. *Magister Ludi (The Glass Bead Game).* New York: Bantam Books, 1972.

———. *Siddhartha.* New York: Bantam Books, 1972.

Hittleman, Richard. *Introduction to Yoga*. New York: Bantam Books, 1969.

Howard, Jane. *Please Touch: A Guided Tour of the Human Potential Movement*. New York: McGraw-Hill Book Co., 1970.

Huang, Al Chung-liang. *Embrace Tiger, Return to Mountain: The Essence of T'ai Chi*. Moab, Utah: Real People Press, 1973.

Hunter, Robert. *The Storming of the Mind: Inside the Consciousness Revolution*. Garden City, N.Y.: Doubleday & Co., Anchor Books, 1972.

Huxley, Aldous. *The Doors of Perception* and *Heaven and Hell*. New York: Harper & Row, 1963.

———. *Island*. New York: Harper & Row, 1972.

———. *The Perennial Philosophy*. New York: Harper & Row, 1970.

Ichazo, Oscar. *The Human Process for Enlightenment and Freedom*. New York: Simon & Schuster, 1976.

Illich, Ivan. *Medical Nemesis: The Expropriation of Health*. New York: Pantheon Books, 1976.

Ingham, Eunice. *Stories the Feet Can Tell: Stepping to Better Health*. Rochester, N.Y.: Eunice D. Ingham, 1959.

———. *Stories the Feet Have Told: Compression Massage*. Rochester, N.Y.: Eunice D. Ingham, 1963.

Iyengar, B. K. S. *Light on Yoga*. New York: Schocken Books, 1973.

Jackson, Jim. *Seeing Yourself See: Eye Exercises for Total Vision*. New York: E. P. Dutton & Co./Saturday Review Press, 1975.

Jacobsen, E. *Progressive Relaxation*. Chicago: University of Chicago Press, 1929.

James, William. *The Varieties of Religious Experience*. New York: Collier Books, 1973.

Janov, Arthur. *The Primal Scream*. New York: Dell Publishing Co., 1971.

Jensen, Bernard. *The Science and Practice of Iridology*. Escondido, Cal.: Bernard Jensen, 1974.

———. *You Can Master Disease*. Solana Beach, Cal.: Bernard Jensen Publishing Co., n.d.

Jonas, Gerald. *Visceral Learning: Toward a Science of Self-Control*. New York: Viking Press, 1973.

Jung, Carl. *Man and His Symbols*. Garden City, N.Y.: Doubleday & Co., 1964.

———. *On the Nature of the Psyche*. Translated by R. F. C. Hull. Princeton, N.J.: Princeton University Press, 1973.

———. *The Portable Jung*. Edited by Joseph Campbell. Translated by R. F. C. Hull. New York: Viking Press, 1972.

———. *Synchronicity: An Acausal Connecting Principle*. Translated by R. F. C. Hull. Princeton, N.J.: Princeton University Press, 1973.

Kapleau, Philip, ed. *The Three Pillars of Zen*. Boston: Beacon Press, 1965.

Kazantzakis, Nikos. *The Last Temptation of Christ*. New York: Bantam Books, 1971.

Keen, Sam. "My New Carnality." *Psychology Today*, October 1970, pp. 59–61.

————. *To a Dancing God.* New York: Harper & Row, 1970.

————. *Voices and Visions.* New York: Harper & Row, 1974.

Keleman, Stanley. *The Human Ground: Sexuality, Self and Survival.* Palo Alto, Cal.: Science and Behavior Books, 1975.

————. *Living Your Dying.* New York: Random House and Berkeley: The Bookworks, 1974.

————. *Your Body Speaks Its Mind: The Bio-energetic Way to Greater Emotional and Sexual Satisfaction.* New York: Simon & Schuster, 1975.

Kelly, C. *New Techniques of Vision Improvement.* Santa Monica, Cal.: Interscience Workshop, 1972.

Kilner, W.J. *The Aura.* New York: Samuel Weiser, 1974.

Koestler, Arthur. *The Act of Creation: A Study of the Conscious and Unconscious in Science and Art.* New York: Dell Publishing Co., 1973.

————. *The Roots of Coincidence: An Excursion into Parapsychology.* New York: Vintage Books, 1972.

Kopp, Sheldon. *Guru: Metaphors from a Psychotherapist.* Palo Alto, Cal.: Science and Behavior Books, 1971.

Kramer, Joel. *The Passionate Mind: A Manual for Living Creatively with One's Self.* Millbrae, Cal.: Celestial Arts, 1974.

Krippner, Stanley. *Song of the Siren.* New York: Harper & Row, 1975.

Krishna, Gopi. *Kundalini, Evolutionary Energy in Man.* Berkeley: Shambala Publications, 1971.

Krishnamurti, J. *Think on These Things.* New York: Harper & Row, 1970.

Kubler-Ross, Elisabeth. *Death: The Final Stage of Growth.* Englewood Cliffs, N.J.: Prentice-Hall, 1975.

Kuhn, Thomas. *The Structure of Scientific Revolutions.* Chicago: University of Chicago Press, 1974.

Kuvalayananda, Swami. *Asanas.* Bombay: Popular Press Private, 1964.

————. *Pranayama.* Bombay: Popular Prakashan, 1972.

Lagerwerff, Ellen B., and Perlroth, Karen A. *Mensendieck Your Posture and Your Pains.* Garden City, N.Y.: Doubleday & Co., Anchor Books, 1973.

Laing, R. D. *The Divided Self.* Baltimore: Penguin Books, 1970.

————. *Knots.* New York: Pantheon Books, 1970.

Lao Tzu. *Tao Te Ching.* Translated by D. C. Lau. Baltimore: Penguin Books, 1963.

————. *Tao Te Ching.* Translated by Gia-Fu Feng and Jane English. New York: Vintage Books, 1972.

————. *The Way of Life According to Lao Tzu.* Translated by Witter Bynner. New York: Capricorn Books, 1962.

Laughingbird. "SAGE." *New Age Journal,* January 1976, pp. 30–33.

Leadbeater, C. W. *The Chakras.* Wheaton, Ill.: Theosophical Publishing House, 1972.

————. *Man Visible and Invisible.* Wheaton, Ill.: Theosophical Publishing House, Inc., 1971.

Leary, Timothy. *Confessions of a Hope Fiend.* New York: Bantam Books, 1973.

————. *The Politics of Ecstasy.* New York: College Notes & Texts, 1968.

Leboyer, Frederick. *Birth Without Violence.* New York: Alfred A. Knopf, 1975.

———. *Loving Hands.* New York: Alfred A. Knopf, 1976.

Le Guin, Ursula. *The Lathe of Heaven.* New York: Avon Books, 1973.

Leonard, George. *Education and Ecstasy.* New York: Dell Publishing Co., 1968.

———. *The Transformation: A Guide to the Inevitable Changes in Humankind.* New York: Dell Publishing Co., 1972.

———. *The Ultimate Athlete.* New York: Viking Press, 1975.

LeShan, Lawrence. *How to Meditate: A Guide to Self-Discovery.* New York: Bantam Books, 1975.

———. *The Medium, the Mystic, and the Physicist.* New York: Ballantine Books, 1975.

Lewis, Howard R., and Lewis, Martha E. *Psychosomatics.* New York: Pinnacle Books, 1975.

Lilly, John. *The Center of the Cyclone: An Autobiography of Inner Space.* New York: Julian Press, 1973.

———. *Programming and Metaprogramming in the Human Biocomputer.* New York: Julian Press, 1972.

———. *Simulations of God: The Science of Belief.* New York: Simon & Schuster, 1975.

Lomi Staff. *The Lomi Papers.* San Francisco: Lomi School Press, 1975.

Lorenz, Konrad. *On Aggression.* New York: Bantam Books, 1969.

Lowen, Alexander. *The Betrayal of the Body.* New York: Collier Books, 1972.

———. *Bioenergetics.* New York: Coward, McCann & Geoghegan, 1975.

———. *Depression and the Body.* Baltimore: Penguin Books, 1973.

———. *The Language of the Body.* New York: Collier Books, 1971.

———. *Love and Orgasm.* London: Staples Press, 1966.

———. *Pleasure—A Creative Approach to Life.* Baltimore: Penguin Books, 1975.

Luce, Gay. *Body Time.* New York: Bantam Books, 1973.

Malinowski, Bronislaw. *Magic, Science and Religion and Other Essays.* New York: Doubleday & Co., Anchor Books, 1964.

Mann, Dr. Felix. *Acupuncture: Cure of Many Diseases.* London: William Clowes & Sons, 1972.

Mar, Timothy. *Face Reading.* New York: Signet Books, 1974.

Marga, Ananda. *Teaching Asanas: An Ananda Marga Manual for Teachers.* Los Altos Hills, Cal.: Ananda Marga Publications, 1973.

Maslow, Abraham. *Religions, Values, and Peak-Experiences.* New York: Viking Press, 1970.

———. *Toward a Psychology of Being.* New York: D. Van Nostrand Co., 1968.

Masters, Robert, and Houston, Jean. *Mind Games: The Guide to Inner Space.* New York: Viking Press, 1972.

———. *The Varieties of Psychedelic Experience.* New York: Dell Publishing Co., 1966.

May, Rollo. *Man's Search for Himself.* New York: W. W. Norton & Co., 1953.

McGuire, Thomas. *The Tooth Trip.* New York: Random House and Berkeley: The Bookworks, 1973.

Meadows, Donella H.; Meadows, Dennis L.; Randers, Jorgen; and Behrens, William. *The Limits to Growth.* New York: Universe Publishers, 1972.

Metzner, Ralph. *Maps of Consciousness.* New York: Collier Books, 1971.

Mishlove, Jeffrey. *The Roots of Consciousness.* New York: Random House and Berkeley: The Bookworks, 1975.

Mishra, Rammurti. *Fundamentals of Yoga.* Garden City, N.Y.: Doubleday & Co., Anchor Books, 1974.

———. *Yoga Sutras: The Textbook of Yoga Psychology.* Garden City, N.Y.: Doubleday & Co., Anchor Books, 1973.

Morehouse, Laurence E., and Gross, Leonard. *Total Fitness.* New York: Pocket Books, 1976.

Moreno, J. L. *Who Shall Survive?* New York: Nervous and Mental Disease Publishing Co., 1934.

Moss, Thelma. *The Probability of the Impossible: Scientific Discoveries and Explorations in the Psychic World.* Los Angeles: J. P. Tarcher, 1974.

Muramoto, Naboru. *Healing Ourselves.* New York: Avon Books, 1973.

Murphy, Gardner. *Human Potentialities.* New York: Viking Press, 1975.

Muses, Charles, and Young, Arthur. *Consciousness and Reality: The Human Pivot Point.* New York: Avon Books, 1974.

Naranjo, Claudio. *The Healing Journey: New Approaches to Consciousness.* New York: Pantheon Books, 1973.

———. *The One Quest.* New York: Ballantine Books, 1973.

———, and Ornstein, Robert. *On the Psychology of Meditation.* New York: Viking Press, 1972.

Needleman, Jacob. *The New Religions.* New York: Pocket Books, 1972.

Neumann, Erich. *The Origins and History of Consciousness.* Princeton, N.J.: Princeton University Press, 1973.

Ornstein, Robert. *The Nature of Human Consciousness: A Book of Readings.* San Francisco: W. H. Freeman & Co., 1973.

———. *The Psychology of Consciousness.* New York: Viking Press, 1973.

Osborn, Arthur. *The Cosmic Womb: An Interpretation of Man's Relationship to the Infinite.* Wheaton, Ill.: Theosophical Publishing House, 1969.

Ostrander, Sheila, and Schroeder, Lynn. *Psychic Discoveries Behind the Iron Curtain.* New York: Bantam Books, 1971.

Otto, Herbert, ed. *Love Today.* New York: Dell Publishing Co., 1972.

Otto, Herbert, and Mann, John. *Ways of Growth: Approaches to Expanding Awareness.* New York: Viking Press, 1968.

Ouspensky, P. D. *In Search of the Miraculous.* New York: Harcourt, Brace & World, 1949.

———. *The Psychology of Man's Possible Evolution.* 2nd ed. New York: Vintage Books, 1974.

Payne, Buryl. *Getting There Without Drugs.* New York: Viking Press, 1973.

Pearce, Joseph. *The Crack in the Cosmic Egg.* New York: Pocket Books, 1973.

————. *Exploring the Crack in the Cosmic Egg: Split Minds and Meta-Realities.* New York: Pocket Books, 1975.

Pelletier, Ken, and Garfield, Charles. *Consciousness East and West.* New York: Harper & Row, 1976.

Perls, Frederick S. *Ego, Hunger and Aggression.* New York: Vintage Books, 1969.

————. *In and Out the Garbage Pail.* Lafayette, Cal.: Real People Press, 1975.

————; Hefferline, Ralph; and Goodman, Paul. *Gestalt Therapy.* New York: Julian Press, 1951.

Pesso, Albert. *Experience in Action: A Psychomotor Psychology.* New York: New York University Press, 1973.

Pirsig, Robert. *Zen and the Art of Motorcycle Maintenance.* New York: Bantam Books, 1975.

Porter, Jean. *Psychic Development.* New York: Random House and Berkeley: The Bookworks, 1974.

Portugal, Pamela. *A Place for Human Beings.* Palo Alto, Cal.: Wild Horses Press, 1974.

Prabhavananda, Swami. *The Song of God: Bhagavad-Gita.* Translated by Christopher Isherwood. New York: New American Library, 1951.

Prestera, Hector, and Kurtz, Ron. *The Body Reveals.* New York: Harper & Row, 1976.

Puharich, Andrija. *Beyond Telepathy.* Garden City, N.Y.: Doubleday & Co., Anchor Books, 1973.

————. *Uri: A Journal of the Mystery of Uri Geller.* New York: Bantam Books, 1975.

Rahula, Walpola. *What the Buddha Taught.* New York: Grove Press, 1962.

Rajneesh, Bhagwan Shree. *Meditation: The Art of Ecstasy.* New York: Harper & Row, 1976.

Raknes, Ola. *Wilhelm Reich and Orgonomy.* Baltimore: Penguin Books, 1971.

Ram Dass, Baba. *The Only Dance There Is.* New York: Doubleday & Co., Anchor Books, 1974.

————. *Remember, Be Here Now.* San Cristobal, N.M.: Lama Foundation, 1971.

Rama, Swami; Ballentine, Rudolph; and Ajaya, Swami. *Yoga and Psychotherapy.* Glenview, Ill.: Himalayan Institute, 1976.

Rampa, T. Lobsang. *The Third Eye.* New York: Ballantine Books, 1972.

Rapoport, Danielle. "Leboyer Follow-up." *The New Age Journal,* January 1976, pp. 14, 15.

Rawson, Philip. *Tantra.* New York: Bounty Books, 1976.

Regush, Nicholas. *The Human Aura.* New York: Berkeley Publishing Corp., 1974.

Reich, Charles. *The Greening of America.* New York: Bantam Books, 1970.
Reich, Wilhelm. *The Cancer Biopathy.* New York: Farrar, Straus & Giroux, 1973.
———. *Character Analysis.* New York: Farrar, Straus & Giroux, 1949.
———. *Cosmic Superimposition.* New York: Farrar, Straus & Giroux, 1973.
———. *The Discovery of the Orgone.* New York: Noonday Press, 1970.
———. *Ether, God and Devil* and *Cosmic Superimposition.* New York: Farrar, Straus & Giroux, 1973.
———. *The Function of the Orgasm.* New York: Farrar, Straus & Cudahy, 1961.
———. *Listen, Little Man!* New York: Noonday Press, 1970.
———. *The Murder of Christ.* New York: Noonday Press, 1972.
———. *Selected Writings: An Introduction to Orgonomy.* New York: Farrar, Straus & Giroux, 1973.
———. *Sex-Pol.* Edited by Lee Baxandall. New York: Vintage Books, 1972.
———. *The Sexual Revolution: Toward a Self-Governing Character Structure.* New York: Farrar, Straus & Giroux, 1969.
Rendel, Peter. *Introduction to the Chakras.* New York: Samuel Weiser, 1974.
Rhine, J. B. *New World of the Mind.* New York: William Morrow & Co., 1973.
———. *The Reach of the Mind.* New York: William Sloan Associates, 1972.
Rhine, Louisa. *Mind Over Matter: Psychokinesis.* New York: Collier Books, 1972.
Roberts, Jane. *The Nature of Personal Reality: A Seth Book.* Englewood Cliffs, N.J.: Prentice-Hall, 1974.
———. *The Seth Material.* Englewood Cliffs, N.J.: Prentice-Hall, 1970.
———. *Seth Speaks—The Eternal Validity of the Soul.* Englewood Cliffs, N.J.: Prentice-Hall, 1972.
Rodale, J. I., and Staff. *Encyclopedia of Common Diseases.* Emmaus, Penn.: Rodale Press, 1974.
Rogers, Carl. *On Encounter Groups.* New York: Harper & Row, 1970.
——— and Stevens, Barry. *Person to Person: The Problem of Being Human.* Lafayette, Cal.: Real People Press, 1974.
Rolf, Ida. *Structural Integration: The Re-Creation of the Balanced Human Body.* New York: Viking Press, 1977.
———. "Structural Integration." *Systematics I,* no. 1 (June 1963).
Rosenberg, Jack. *Total Orgasm.* New York: Random House and Berkeley: The Bookworks, 1973.
Rubin, Jerry. *Growing (Up) at 37.* New York: M. Evans & Co., 1976.
Rush, Anne Kent. *Getting Clear: Body Work for Women.* New York: Random House and Berkeley: The Bookworks, 1973.
Samuels, Michael, and Bennett, Harold. *The Well Body Book.* New York: Random House and Berkeley: The Bookworks, 1973.

Samuels, Michael, and Samuels, Nancy. *Seeing with the Mind's Eye.* New York: Random House and Berkeley: The Bookworks, 1975.

Satchidananda, Swami Yogiraj. *Integral Yoga Hatha.* New York: Holt, Rinehart & Winston, 1970.

Schoop, Trudy, and Mitchell, Peggy. *Won't You Join the Dance?* Mayfield Publishing Co., 1974.

Schutz, William. *Elements of Encounter.* Big Sur, Cal.: Joy Press, 1973.

————. *Here Comes Everybody.* New York: Harper & Row, 1971.

————. *Joy—Expanding Human Awareness.* New York: Grove Press, 1968.

———— and Turner, Evelyn. *Evy.* New York: Harper & Row, 1976.

Selye, Hans. *The Stress of Life.* New York: McGraw-Hill Book Co., 1956.

————. *Stress Without Distress.* Philadelphia: J. B. Lippincott & Co., 1974.

Shah, Idries. *Caravan of Dreams.* Baltimore: Penguin Books, 1968.

————. *Tales of the Dervishes.* New York: E.P. Dutton & Co., 1967.

Sharma, Pandit. *Yoga for Backaches.* New York: Cornerstone Library, 1971.

Sheldon, W. H. *Atlas of Men: A Guide For Somatotyping the Adult Male at all Ages.* New York: Harper & Row, 1954.

————; Stevens, S. S.; and Tucker, W. B. *The Varieties of Human Physique.* New York: Harper & Row, 1940.

Shuman, David, and Staab, George. *Your Aching Back.* New York: Gramercy Publishing Co., 1976.

Silverberg, Robert. *Son of Man.* New York: Ballantine Books, 1971.

Sinclair. *Mental Radio.* New York: Collier Books, 1971.

Sivananda, Sri. *Gyana Yoga.* Delhi: Motilal Banarsidass, 1973.

Skinner, B. F. *Beyond Freedom and Dignity.* New York: Alfred A. Knopf, 1971.

Smith, Adam. *Powers of Mind.* New York: Random House, 1975.

Smith, Wilfred. *The Meaning and End of Religion.* New York: New American Library, 1964.

Soleri, Paolo. *The Bridge Between Matter and Spirit Is Matter Becoming Spirit.* Garden City, N.Y.: Doubleday & Co., Anchor Books, 1973.

Spangler, David. *Revelation: The Birth of a New Age.* Moray, Scotland: Findhorn Foundation, 1974.

Stapleton, Olaf. *Last and First Men: A Story of the Near and Far Future* and *Star Maker.* New York: Dover Publications, 1968.

Stearn, Jess. *Yoga, Youth, and Reincarnation.* New York: Bantam Books, 1971.

Steiner, Rudolf. *Knowledge of the Higher Worlds and Its Attainment.* New York: Anthroposophic Press, 1947.

Stephen. *The Caravan.* New York: Random House and Berkeley: The Bookworks, 1972.

————. *Monday Night Class.* Santa Rosa, Cal.: Book Farm, 1970.

Stevens, John. *Awareness: Exploring, Experimenting, Experiencing.* New York: Bantam Books, 1973.

Stonehouse, Dr. Bernard. *The Way Your Body Works.* New York: Crown Publishers, 1974.

Subramuniya, Master. *Raja Yoga.* San Francisco: Comstock House, 1973.

Suzuki, Shunryu. *Zen Mind, Beginner's Mind.* New York: Walker/Weatherhill, 1970.

Sweigard, Lulu. *Human Movement Potential.* New York: Harper & Row, 1974.

Tart, Charles, ed. *Altered States of Consciousness: A Book of Readings.* New York: John Wiley & Sons, 1969.

Teilhard de Chardin, Pierre. *Building the Earth.* New York: Avon Books, 1970.

———. *The Phenomenon of Man.* New York: Harper & Row, 1965.

Terwilliger, Robert. *Meaning and Mind: A Study in the Psychology of Language.* New York: Oxford University Press, 1968.

Thompson, Clem. *Manual of Structural Kinesiology.* St. Louis: C. V. Mosby Co., 1969.

Thompson, William Irwin. *At the Edge of History: Speculations on the Transformation of Culture.* New York: Harper & Row, 1972.

———. *Passages About Earth: An Exploration of the New Planetary Culture.* New York: Harper & Row, 1974.

Todd, Mabel. *The Thinking Body: A Study of the Balancing Forces of Dynamic Man.* Brooklyn, N.Y.: Dance Horizons, 1973.

Toffler, Alvin. *Future Shock.* New York: Bantam Books, 1972.

Tompkins, Peter, and Bird, Christopher. *The Secret Life of Plants.* New York: Avon Books, 1973.

Trungpa, Chogyam. *Cutting Through Spiritual Materialism.* Berkeley: Shambala Publications, 1973.

———. *Meditation in Action.* Berkeley: Shambala Publications, 1969.

——— and Guenther, Herbert. *The Dawn of Tantra.* Berkeley: Shambala Publications, 1975.

Tulku, Tarthang. *Reflections of Mind.* California: Dharma Publishing, 1975.

Van Vliet, C. J. *The Coiled Serpent.* Los Angeles: De Vorss & Co., 1959.

Vishnudevananda, Swami. *The Complete Illustrated Book of Yoga.* New York: Pocket Books, 1972.

Vonnegut, Kurt. *The Sirens of Titan.* New York: Dell Publishing Co., 1974.

Watts, Alan. *Beyond Theology: The Art of Godmanship.* New York: Vintage Books, 1973.

———. *The Book . . .* New York: Vintage Books, 1972.

———. *In My Own Way: An Autobiography.* New York: Vintage Books, 1973.

———. *The Joyous Cosmology.* New York: Vintage Books, 1970.

———. *Psychotherapy East and West.* New York: Ballantine Books, 1969.

———. *This Is It and Other Essays.* New York: Collier Books, 1967.

Weed, Joseph. *Wisdom of the Mystic Masters.* West Nyack, N.Y.: Parker Publishing Co., 1972.

Weil, Andrew. *The Natural Mind: A New Way of Looking at Drugs and the Higher Consciousness.* Boston: Houghton Mifflin Co., 1972.

White, John. *The Highest State of Consciousness.* Garden City, N.Y.: Doubleday & Co., Anchor Books, 1972.

Wilhelm, Richard. *The I Ching: Book of Changes.* Princeton, N.J.: Princeton University Press, 1950.

Wilson, Colin. *The Mind Parasites.* Oakland, Cal.: Oneiric Press, 1972.

————. *New Pathways in Psychology: Maslow and the Post-Freudian Revolution.* New York: New American Library, 1974.

Wolff, Charlotte. *The Hand in Psychological Diagnosis.* New Delhi: Sagar Publications, 1972.

Woodruff, Sir John. *The Serpent Power.* Madras: Ganesh & Col, 1918.

Wyckoff, James. *Wilhelm Reich: Life Force Explorer.* Greenwich, Conn.: Fawcett Publications, 1973.

Yogananda, Paramahansa. *Autobiography of a Yogi.* Los Angeles: Self Realization Fellowship, 1969.

INDEX

abdominal cavity, 119–127, 131–137; tension in, and pelvis, 83–85
access, future/past, 241
aggressiveness, 134–135
Aikido, 58
Ajna (6th chakra), 89, 91, 186, 204, 216; and expanded mental powers, 238–243
ambidextrousness, 33–34
Anahata (4th chakra), 87, 90, 148
anal region, 85, 91–95; blockage of, 95–98
Anderson, Walt, 102
anger: and back/front split, 41–43; and diaphragm, 141; and jaw tension, 196–197; and tension headaches, 236–237; and upper back, 14, 180–185
ankles, 64–65; sprained, 21, 38
anxiety: and chest expansion, 162; and shallow breathing, 146–147
arms, 170–180; fat, underdeveloped, 174; left, 39; massive, overmuscled, 174; and nonverbal communication, 178–180; right, 39; thin,

tight, 174; weak, underdeveloped, 173–174
arthritis, 38, 170
asthma, 21, 72, 154; and chest contraction, 157; and pelvis position, 85; and top/bottom split, 38. *See also* breathing
astral travel, 241
auras, reading of, 241
awkwardness, and top/bottom split, 38

"baby eyes," 225–226
back, lower, 137–140; and anal-region holding, 96, 97; as mediator, 138; and pelvis position, 83, 84; and upper back pain, 139
back, upper, 180–185; and anger, 14; and lower back pain, 138–140
Baker, Elsworth, 93–94, 142; on eyes, 223
balance, sense of, 222–223
being/doing split, 44–46
belly, 122–127, 131–137; internal func-

tioning of, 131–134; nervous, 38, 132, 142; and top/bottom split, 38

bhaktiyoga, 66

bioenergetics, 9–10, 15, 84, 110, 117, 136, 244, 253

biofeedback, 15, 244, 253; and migraine headaches, 45

"birthwithoutviolence," 33–34

bladdertrouble, 83

Boadella, David, 110, 165

bodyarmor, 103

"body expression," and "character," 9–10

Body Language (Fast), 179

body-reading process, 3–10, 15

bodymind: changes in, 58–60, 129–131, 177–178, 263–264; and emotions, 122–125; formation components of, 20–26; major splits in, 26–46; mapping of, 28–29; "masculine/feminine," 29–32; self-creation of, 39–40; self-examination of, 26–29; and self-realization, 256–264

bodymind splits, 26–29; front/back, 40–43; head/body, 43–44; right /left, 29–34; top/bottom, 34–40; torso/limbs, 44–46

brain activity, right/left, 29

breasts, 154

breathing: chest contraction and, 155–159; and diaphragm, 140–143; and lungs, 145–148; of older people, 147–148; shallow, 146–147; and shoulder position, 169; and stuttering, 202–203; and throat, 195

bronchitis, 72, 154; and chest contraction, 157; and pelvis position, 85

brow (forehead), 236–238

brow (frontal) chakra (Ajna), 89, 91, 186, 204, 216; and expanded mental powers, 238–243

bruxion, 196

buck teeth, 196

Bucke, Richard M., 258–262

Campbell, Joseph, 120, 258

canalis centralis, 86

chakra(s), 86–91; brow, 89, 91, 186, 204, 216, 238–243; crown, 89, 186, 204, 256–262; heart, 87, 90, 148; navel, 87, 90, 120; progression through, 89–91; root, 87, 92, 120; spleen, 87, 90, 98, 120; throat, 87, 186, 187, 195, 203–215

changes: in bodymind, 58–60; physical and emotional, 129–131, 177–178, 262–264

character: and "body expression," 9–10; and sexuality, 102

"character armor," 102–103, 165

charge stage, of orgasm cycle, 104–105

chest cavity, 144–162; chest colds, 72, 85, 154, 157; contraction of, 155–159, 168; expansion of, 159–162, 168; heart, 148–153, 155; lungs, 145–148; and neglect, 14; self-examination of, 154–155

"chi" energy, 61

childbirth, and handedness, 33–34

chin. *See* jaw

chiropractic, 86, 181

clairvoyance, 241

clutching feet, 54–56

coccygeal vertebra, 80

cold hands, 173, 175–177

colds, 72, 154; and chest contraction, 157; and pelvis position, 85

communication, 187; nonverbal, 178–180

compulsives, and lower back pain, 140

consciousness: cosmic, 258, 259–262; evolution of, 258–262; self-, 259–261; simple, 260–261

coordination, and top/bottom split, 38

cosmic consciousness, 258, 259–262

Cosmic Consciousness (Bucke), 258–262

coughing, 195

creativity, and right side, 30

crown (coronal) chakra (Sahasrara), 89, 186, 204; and self-realization, 256–262 crying styles, and right/left preferences, 31

deafness, 218–223
death, expression of emotion over, 198–199
depression, 22; and chest contraction, 162
diabetes, 142
diaphragm, 140–143; pelvic, 93, 97; and stuttering, 202–203
dis-ease. *See* injury and dis-ease
discharge stage, of orgasm cycle, 104, 105–106
divining, 241
Dychtwald, Ken: at Esalen, 10–16; on expanding limits, 212–215; faces of, 217–218; and flat feet, 53, 59–60; heart/love experience of, 150–153; identity crisis of, 205–209; and knee trouble, 65–74; physical description of, 18–20; Pierrakos and, 3–9; and Rolfing, 125–127, 128–131; on sexuality, 115–118; and T'ai Chi, 47–50; and yoga, 65–74
Dychtwald, Mrs., 132–133
Dychtwald, Seymour, 160–161, 213–215

ears, 220–223; and balance, 223
Eastern cultures, holistic approach of, 24
"edge" concept, of yoga, 67–69, 113, 130–131
ego: and head position, 194; and shoulder position, 168
eliminative disorders, 84, 93–96
emotions: in the abdomen, 122–127, 131–137; arms and hands and, 170–180; and bodymind, 20–22, 24, 122–125; and chest cavity, 144–145, 154–155; and chest contraction, 156–159; and chest expansion, 159–162; and diaphragm, 140–143; expression of, 122–125, 132; and eye dysfunctions, 226–231; and eye shape, 224–226; and facial masks, 216–219; and hearing, 220–222; and injury and disease, 124, 132–137; in neck area, 189–195; "negative," 40–43; and ocular segment, 216–238; and oral area, 195–203; and physical change, 129–131, 177–178, 262–264; physical consolidation of, 11–13; and right/left preferences, 30–33; and shoulders, 164–170; and upper back, 181–185
emphysema, 154
encounter groups, 11, 15, 110, 244, 253, 254
enlightenment, 258; and cosmic consciousness, 261–262
environment, and bodymind formation, 20, 23
Esalen Institute (Big Sur, Calif.), 10, 30, 134
EST, 243
evolution, of consciousness, 258–262
excitation stage, of orgasm cycle, 105
extrasensory perception, 240–243
eyes, 223–236; "baby," 225–226; bulging, 225; deep-set, 225; farsightedness of, 231; hard, 226; iridology and, 231–236; large, rounded, 224; left, 31; nearsightedness of, 226–231; right, 31; sclerology and, 231; self-examination of, 223–224; shapes of, 224–226; soft, 226

face, 216–220
farsightedness, 231
Fast, Julius, on touching, 179–180
fear: and back/front split, 42–43; and shoulder positions, 164–165, 167–168
feelings. *See* emotions

feet, 51–63, 172; clutching, 54–56; flat, 38, 52–54, 59–60; healthy, 52; lead, 58; tiptoers, 57; weight on heels of, 56–57; and zone therapy, 60–63
Feldenkrais, Moshe, 209
Feldenkrais method, 15, 110, 117, 139, 243, 253; self-image and, 209–212
feminine. *See* masculine/feminine aspects
flat feet, 38, 52–54, 59–60
fondling, as nonverbal communication, 179–180
foot reflexology, 60–63
forehead, 236–238
foreplay, 105
Freud, Sigmund, 94, 101, 103
front/back split, 40–43
"frozen history," 165
future access, 241

gall bladder disease, 142
genital region, 98–100. *See also* sexuality
Gerrard, Eugenia, 148
Gestalt therapy, 15, 110, 253
gluteus maximus, contraction of, 96
gravity, and bodymind, 129
grounding: and feet, 52, 59–60; legs and, 50, 74–78; and top/bottom split, 34

"habit patterns," 11–12
hamstring muscles, 78, 97
hands, 170, 171; cold, 173, 175–177; and nonverbal communication, 178–180; right/left, 32–34
hate, arms and hands and, 172
hatha yoga, 67
head: forward position of, 193; positions of, 193–195; side-leaning positions of, 194. *See also specific parts of the head*
head/body split, 43–44

headaches: migraine, 45; tension, 38, 83, 236–237
healing, 15, 241
hearing, 220–223
heart, 148–153, 155; and chest cavity, 155, 162
heart (cardiac) chakra (Anahata), 87, 90, 148
hemorrhoids, 22, 96; and pelvis position, 83, 84
heredity, and bodymind formation, 20
high blood pressure, 162
hips. *See* pelvis
human-potential movement, 243–255; meditation and, 246–253, 254; reasons for, 244–245; techniques of, 253–255. *See also specific approaches*
Huxley, Aldous, 242
hyperopia, 231
hypertension, 162

Ichazo, Oscar, 173
Ida (energy channel), 86
impulsives, and lower back pain, 140
injury and dis-ease, 6–7; attentiveness to, 177–178; and diaphragm, 141–143; of ears, 220–223; and emotional blockage, 124–125, 132–137; of eyes, 223, 226–231; iris diagnosis of, 231–236; sclera diagnosis of, 231, 236; and stress, 65–74; and top/bottom split, 38; and yoga, 66–74. *See also specific body parts and maladies*
intellect, and emotions, 124–125
intuition, 240
iridology, 231–236

jaw, 195–215; clenched, 201; protruding, 201; receding, 201; and sadness, 14
Jensen, Bernard, on iridology, 231–233

jnana (gnani) yoga, 66
Johnson, Virginia, 110
joints, 64–65, 170, 172

Kairos (Rancho Santa Fe, Calif.), 9
karma yoga, 66
Keleman, Stanley, 9
Kinsey, Alfred, 110
knees, 64–65
Kramer, Joel, on meditation, 248
Kundalini energy, 85–86, 113, 120
Kundalini yoga, 67, 85–95

lead feet, 58
Leboyer, Frederick, 33–34
left side, 30–34; head tilted to, 194; of shoulders, 148, 155, 168, 170
legs, 74–78, 172; backs of, 77–78, 140; fat, underdeveloped, 75–76; left/right, 39; massive, overmuscled, 76; and pelvis position, 84; and T'ai Chi, 48–50; thin, tight, 76–77; weak, underdeveloped, 75
libido, 103
lisp, and jaw tension, 196
liver conditions, 142
lordosis, 141
lost objects, location of, 241
love: arms and hands and, 171–172; and hearts, 150–153
Lowen, Alexander, 9, 10, 80, 87, 138; on brow positions, 237; on face, 216–217; on head positions, 194; on top/bottom split, 37
lower back. *See* back, lower
lungs, 145–148
lymphatic system, and foot reflexology, 61

Maithuna (tantric lovemaking), 111–115
Manipura (3rd chakra), 87, 90, 120
mantric meditation, 250
masculine/feminine aspects: right/left

split and, 30–31; of shoulders, 170. *See also* left side; right side
Maslow, Abraham, 248
massage, 15; of the foot, 61; Rolfing as, 12–13
masseter muscle, 195–196
Masters, William, 110
meditation, 15, 246–253, 254; aspects of, 252–253; T'ai Chi as, 48–49
meridians, and foot reflexology, 61
migraine headaches, 45
mind/body dualism, 5–8; in Western cultures, 24–25
moral exaltation, and cosmic consciousness, 261–262
motion, and flat feet, 53–54
Muladhara (1st chakra), 87, 91–92, 120
myopia, 226–231

Nature of Personal Reality, The: A Seth Book (Roberts), 134–135
nausea, 142
navel (umbilical) chakra (Manipura), 87, 90, 120
nearsightedness, 226–231
neck, 187–195; long, 194; as mediator, 189–193, 194; positions of, 193–195; self-examination of, 187–189; stout, 194
nervousness, 22. *See also* anxiety
neuromuscular patterns, breaking up of, 209–212
neurosis, and sexual dysfunction, 101–102, 109
nonverbal communication, 178–180
nutrition, and bodymind formation, 20, 23

ocular segment, 216–255; ears, 220–223; eyes, 223–236; forehead, 236–238; psychoemotional dynamics in, 216–238; spiritual aspects of, 238–255
older people: breathing of, 147–148;

hearing of, 221–223; sexuality of, 107–109
oral segment, 195–215; psychoemotional dynamics in, 195–203; spiritual aspects of, 203–215
orgasm: Reichian view of, 101–106, 109; in tantric yoga, 111, 113–115
orgasm cycle, 104–107, 109
"orgastic potency," 102, 103, 109
orgastic reflex, 105–106
orgone, 103, 109, 145
Ornstein, Robert, 30
ovarian cysts, 72
overbite, 196

paranoia, and shoulder position, 168
past access, 241
peak experiences, 248
pectoral muscles, 154, 155
pelvic diaphragm, 93, 97
pelvis, 80–118; anal region of, 85, 91–98; downward-tipped, 83–85; genital region of, 14, 98–100; and lower back pain, 133–140; positioning of, 80–81; self-examination of, 79–80; upward-tipped, 81–83
perception, expanded, 238–243
Perls, Fritz, on anxiety, 146–147
physical activity, and bodymind formation, 20–21
physiognomy, 220
Pierrakos, John, 3–5, 8, 9, 10
pineal gland, 258
Pingala (energy channel), 86
pituitary gland, 258
plateau stage, of orgasm cycle, 105, 106
prana, 145, 153
prana yoga, 67
pranayama, 66, 145
precognition, 241
Prestera, Hector, 10, 12, 181–184, 198
primal therapy, 110
privacy: and front/back split, 40–43; and top/bottom split, 34–36, 38

psychedelicism, 15
psychic senses, 238–243
psychodrama, 15, 198
psychokinesis, 241
psychometry, 241
"pushovers," 56–57

raja yoga, 66
Rajneesh meditation, 250
Rapoport, Danielle, 33–34
rationality, and brow tension, 236–237
Raynaud's disease, 175–177
recovery phase, of orgasm cycle, 105, 106
Reich, Wilhelm, 9, 87, 93; on arms, 174; on diaphragm, 141; and sexuality, 101–107, 109–111, 114–115
Reichian energetics, 15, 86, 137, 253
relaxation stage, of orgasm cycle, 104, 105–106
release stage, of orgasm cycle, 105, 106
resonance, emotional, 13–14
responsibility: and bodymind, 263–264; and neck area, 189–190; and shoulder position, 14, 167
retrocognition, 241
right side, 29–33; head tilted to, 194
Roberts, Jane, 134–135
Rolf, Ida, 11, 80, 129
Rolfing, 11–15, 86, 110, 117, 243, 253, 254; Dychtwald and, 125–127; and heart area, 148–150; as three processes, 127–131
root chakra (Muladhara), 87, 91–92, 120
Rosenberg, Jack, 104

sacral vertebra, 80
SAGE Project, 107–108, 147–148, 222
Sahasrara (7th chakra), 89, 187, 204; self-realization and, 256–262
Schutz, William, 10, 13, 21, 196; on breathing, 142–143; on chakras,

90–91; on feet, 53–56; on oral area, 195–196; on right/left split, 31–32

sciatica, 72

sclerology, 231, 236

self-awareness, heightened, 238–243; and human-potential movement, 243–255

"self-consciousness," 260–261

self-development, and human-potential movement, 243–255

self-identification, 187, 203–215

self-image, Feldenkrais and, 209–212

self-realization, 256–264; and body-mind, 256–258, 262–264; and cosmic consciousness, 259–262

semicircular canals, 223

senility, 222

senses, psychic, 238–243

sensory awareness, 15, 110, 244

sexual dysfunction, 72; and anal-region holding, 97; and genital region, 98–100; and neurosis, 101–102, 109–111; and pelvis position, 83; Reichian view of, 101–107, 109–111; and top/bottom split, 38

sexual role. *See* masculine/feminine aspects

sexuality: conflicts about, 115–118; of older people, 107–109; and pelvis position, 14, 81–85; Reichian view of, 101–107, 109–111, 114; tantric yoga and, 111–115

shallow breathing, and anxiety, 146–147

Shiatsu, 15

shoulders, 14, 163–170; bowed, rounded, 167; forward, hunched, 168–169; left/right, 148, 155, 166, 170; raised, 167–168; retracted, pulled-back, 170; self-examination of, 163–164; square, 168

Show Me How You Breathe and I Will Tell You How You Live (movie), 148

siddha yoga, 67

"simple consciousness," 260–261

sore throat, 21

spastic colon, 72, 132

sphincter muscles, 91–94

spine, and emotions, 181–185. *See also* back, lower; back, upper

spirituality: of ocular segment, 238–255; of oral area, 203–215

spleen (splenic) chakra (Svadhisthana), 87, 90, 98, 120

stress, and injury, 65–74

structural integration. *See* Rolfing

stuttering, 202–203

Sushumna (energy conduit), 86

Svadhisthana (2nd chakra), 87, 90, 98, 120

T'ai Chi, 47–50, 58, 250, 253

"tan tien" (body's center), 48, 49

tantric yoga, 67, 85, 100; and sexuality, 111–115

Taoism, 47

teeth, grinding of, 196

telepathy, 241

tension headaches, 38, 83, 236–237

tension stage, of orgasm cycle, 104, 105

third eye. *See* Ajna

Thompson, William Irwin, 111

thoracic segment, 144–152; chest contraction in, 155–159; chest expansion in, 159–162; heart, 148–153, 155; lungs, 145–148; self-examination of, 154–155

throat, 195–215. *See also* neck

throat (laryngeal) chakra (Vishuddha), 87–88, 186, 187, 195; and self-identification, 203–215

tiptoers, 57

toilet training, 93–95

Tommy (rock opera), 219

top/bottom split, 34–40; large top, small bottom, 36–37; small top, large bottom, 36

torso/limbs split, 44–46; strong torso, weak limbs, 45; weak torso, strong limbs, 45–46

Total Orgasm (Rosenberg), 104–106

touching, as nonverbal communication, 178–180
transcendental meditation, 243, 250
"trust" exercise, 77–78
tuberculosis, 162

ulcers: intestinal, 132; peptic, 142
upper back. *See* back, upper

varicose veins, 38
vibrational empathy, 241
Vipassasa meditation, 250
Vishuddha (5th chakra), 87–88, 186, 187, 195; and self-identification, 203–215
voice, and throat area, 195, 198
vomiting, after Rolfing, 127

Weaver, Judith, 47, 49
Western cultures, mind/body dualism in, 24–25
Who, The, 219
Wilhelm Reich: The Evolution of His Work (Boadella), 165
Wilson, Chet, 125–126

yin/yang, 30
yoga, 16, 48, 49, 117, 243, 250, 253; and "edge" concept, 67–68, 113, 130–131; health and, 66–74; Kundalini, 67, 85–95; tantric, 67, 85, 100, 111–115; types of, 67

zazen meditation, 250–251
zone therapy, 60–63

ABOUT THE AUTHOR

Ken Dychtwald, Ph.D., is a psychologist, gerontologist, lecturer, author, and outspoken figure
in the fields of bodymind development, wellness,
and human aging.

Presently, he is president of a seminar and
training company, Dychtwald & Associates, and
president of a consulting firm, Age Wave, Inc.
in Berkeley, California. Ken was the founding
director of the "Institute on Aging, Health and
Work" of the Washington Business Group on
Health. He is the director of the Bodymind
Training Institute of Scandinavia; and serves as
senior advisor for the Task Force on Aging
Studies, El Camino Hospital, Mountain View,
California.

In his capacity as an authority on wellness and
health promotion he has consulted with and/or
designed programs for a variety of corporations,
health facilities, and government agencies in-

cluding: ABC Television, American Association of Retired Persons (AARP), A.T.& T., Bank of America, Blue Cross/Blue Shield, Office of Technology Assessment, U.S. Congress, Panasonic Company, The United States Commission on Aging, United States Department of Agriculture, and Upjohn Health Care Services

Dr. Dychtwald is also an adjunct instructor in psychology, gerontology, and health-related sciences at several colleges and universities, and frequently appears on television and radio shows throughout North America including Good Morning America, the Merv Griffin Show, CBS Morning, A.M. Los Angeles, and A.M. San Francisco.

In addition to *Bodymind* (translated into nine foreign languages), his publications include: *Millennium: Glimpses into the 21st Century* (translated into three foreign languages), *Stress-Management: Take Charge of Your Life, Wellness and Health Promotion for the Elderly, The Aging of America* (forthcoming), and more than one hundred articles in professional journals and popular magazines.